Clinician's Guide to the
Twelve Step Principles

Notice

Medicine is an ever changing science. As new research and clinical experience broaden our knowledge, changes in treatment and drug therapy are required. The authors and the publisher of this work have checked with sources believed to be reliable in their efforts to provide information that is complete and generally in accord with the standards accepted at the time of publication. However, in view of the possibility of human error or changes in medical sciences, neither the authors nor the publisher nor any other party who has been involved in the preparation or publication of this work warrants that the information contained herein is in every respect accurate or complete, and they disclaim all responsibility for any errors or omissions or for the results obtained from use of the information contained in this work. Readers are encouraged to confirm the information contained herein with other sources. For example and in particular, readers are advised to check the product information sheet included in the package of each drug they plan to administer to be certain that the information contained in this work is accurate and that changes have not been made in the recommended dose or in the contraindications for administration. This recommendation is of particular importance in connection with new or infrequently used drugs.

Clinician's Guide to the
Twelve Step Principles

Marvin D. Seppala, M.D.

McGraw-Hill
Medical Publishing Division

New York Chicago San Francisco Lisbon London Madrid Mexico City
Milan New Delhi San Juan Seoul Singapore Sydney Toronto

McGraw-Hill

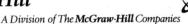

A Division of The **McGraw·Hill** Companies

1 2 3 4 5 6 7 8 9 0 DOC DOC 0 9 8 7 6 5 4 3 2 1

ISBN 0-07-134718-6

This book was set in Korinna by Keyword Publishing Services.
The editor was Martin Wonsiewicz.
The production supervisor was Catherine Saggese.
Project management was provided by Keyword Publishing Services.
The cover design was by Aimee Nordin.
R.R. Donnelley & Sons was the printer and binder.

This book is printed on acid-free paper.

Library of Congress Cataloging-in-Publication Data
Seppala, Marvin D.
    Clinician's guide to the Twelve Step principles / author, Marvin D. Seppala.
        p. ;   cm.
    Includes bibliographical references and index.
    ISBN 0-07-134718-6
        1. Substance abuse—Patients—Rehabilitation.   2. Twelve-step programs.   3. Recovering
    addicts.   4. Substance abuse—Treatment.   5. Psychotherapy.   I. Title: Clinician's guide to
    the Twelve Step principles.   II. Title: Twelve Step principles.   III. Title
        [DNLM: 1. Substance-Related Disorders—rehabilitation.   2. Behavior,
    Addictive—therapy.   3. Psychotherapy.   WM 270 S479 2001]
    RC564.S47 2001
    616.86'06—dc21   00-049629

Contents

Preface

Academic efforts to address alcoholism and addiction seldom emphasize the Twelve Steps. Twelve Step programs are the most widely attended and successful methods of addressing the addictions, but gain little attention in the professional literature. These programs remain misunderstood, ignored, and sometimes even mocked, in spite of broad appeal and documented performance. There are over 98,000 A.A. groups worldwide representing 171 different countries and territories. Significant improvement in all measures of drinking problems was noted by Humphreys at one-year follow-up of untreated individuals attending A.A. No research has revealed a method of addressing the addictions that is significantly superior to the Twelve Steps. The "best" attempts at research-based therapies, interventions, and treatment methods have yet to prove more successful than a spiritual program initiated by two desperate alcoholics in 1935.

While other branches of medicine are examining the roles of "alternative" therapies, including prayer and meditation, the academic emphasis in addiction has not embraced such an inquiry into these established programs. Controversy illuminates the very essence of these programs; they feature spiritual discipline in healing chronic illness. It is my hope that the reader can withhold judgment and bias as it relates to this spiritual approach, thus gaining an opportunity to examine a fascinating and remarkably successful method of healing.

These programs have grown dramatically worldwide without professional input or scientific inquiry. I have attempted to describe the Twelve Steps as they are actually practiced, without providing a psychiatric explanation. It is my hope that this approach will provide clinicians with a knowledge base familiar to members participating in these programs, thus allowing for individual interpretation and the ability to readily communicate a working knowledge of the Steps. Expression of this knowledge will engage members of these programs who can become our greatest teachers.

REFERENCE

K. Humphreys, R. H. Moos, and C. Cohen, Social and community resources and long-term recovery from treated and untreated alcoholism. *Journal of Studies on Alcohol*, 1997, 58:231–238.

Acknowledgments

It is impossible to acknowledge many of the people contributing to the ideas expressed in this book, because so much is taken directly from Twelve Step meetings. They remain anonymous, working their programs and sharing themselves freely with others. I am indebted to them for taking me in and teaching me about this incredible, spiritual program of recovery. I have also learned from the people who have come to me for psychiatric care while they have been working Twelve Step programs, and thank them for the privilege of sharing in their journeys.

I discussed the basic concepts of the Steps with several friends who generously contributed their thoughts and feelings about recovery. The Twelve Steps are a verbal tradition, shared by telling one's "story," and they provided examples of this profound adventure in growth and healing. They also supported me, and encouraged my efforts at describing the Twelve Steps without defining those concepts purposefully left for individual interpretation. I am particularly grateful for the opportunity to discuss spirituality with people who recognize the necessity of conscious attention to the practice of spiritual principles in daily life. Thus, a special thanks to Dave C., Tom K., Doug L., Cheryl M., Dick M., Pat S., and Jon W.

I continue to be inspired and supported by two medical classmates. I am appreciative of Keith Berge's deeply thoughtful approach to life, and motivated by his consistent efforts to challenge himself. Paul Dart provided a needed perspective with very little effort, a wonderful example of his insightful nature.

I must thank everyone at Hazelden who has helped me over the years. I am grateful to Hazelden Publishing and McGraw-Hill for trusting this task to a first-time author. I owe a special thanks to Gary Hestness for his friendship and his role in this project. The editor, Steve Leyman, is an old friend and played an integral role, sharing ideas and the excitement of creation.

I would like to thank friends and neighbors for their important roles in my life, especially in understanding the effort required to complete this text. Thank you, Doug, for keeping me sane with intermittent, joyous, excursions in the great state of Oregon.

My family is excited about this book, and a bit tired of the extracurricular effort it required. They have supported me through-out, and graciously contributed when I was preoccupied. Linda, my wife and soulmate, consistently encourages my efforts; her love influences everything I do.

M.D.S.

Clinician's Guide to the
Twelve Step Principles

Introduction

More people use Twelve Step programs than any other method to address addictive disease, yet little information about these programs has been written for professionals. Academic and research efforts in addiction emphasize neurochemistry and behavioral models, but tend to ignore the Twelve Steps that have been successfully assisting alcoholics for the past sixty years. These programs are the most likely to be used by the clinician faced with addictive disease, and certainly the most likely recovery programs to be represented in the community. This text is intended to provide information about the Twelve Steps for clinicians faced with this prevalent disease.

This is a reference text designed to furnish essential information about Twelve Step programs, featuring the individual Steps. These programs provide limited written information with basic textbooks, which are extremely useful to the interested clinician. They are based on a verbal tradition, thus most of the information needed by individual members is obtained by participating in meetings and communicating with more experienced members. These factors have limited the information available to clinicians. This text was developed using information gathered from the textbooks of several Twelve Step programs, clinical practice in the field of addiction medicine, and most importantly attending Twelve Step meetings and having discussions with members. Definitions are lacking in the available written works, and members avoid them, usually deferring to the individual's conceptualization. The verbal tradition is founded on members "telling their stories," which emphasize how they handled issues or problems using the program and specific Steps. This text treats the principles of the Twelve Steps in a similar manner, thus specific definitions are lacking and most information is highly interpretable. A specific attempt has been made to avoid providing definition where it does not exist in actual practice. The Twelve Steps, like the individuals using them, are a work in progress, and exist as a living, transformational process. As such, this is a unique interpretation, based on multiple resources, intended to provide clinicians with information that will enhance their ability to care for clients in the midst of active addiction as well as members of Twelve Step programs.

The text provides detailed information about each particular Step, which can be used to gain a comprehensive understanding of the program or examined individually when discussing a particular aspect of recovery with a member. The individual Steps are representative of any Twelve Step program (Alcoholics Anonymous, Narcotics Anonymous ...), except for the First Step which references a particular type of addiction. Thus, a thorough understanding of the Steps translates to all of the Twelve Step programs. Information for this text was collected from several Twelve Step programs, with a preponderance from A.A. since the Twelve Steps originated with A.A., and the others use A.A.'s description as a foundation for their own programs. The structure and basic functioning of Twelve Step programs is described, providing the clinician with a general model of Twelve Step meetings. It would be tremendously beneficial for the clinician interested in these programs to attend meetings for an authentic, firsthand examination.

Due to the prevalence of the addictive disorders all clinicians should have a working knowledge of the Twelve Steps. Coexisting medical and psychological conditions result in regular care of Twelve Step members by most clinicians, whether they take an interest in addiction or not. Knowledge of Twelve Step programs can enhance treatment efforts, and prevent mistakes. The information provided in this text will help equip clinicians to treat members of Twelve Step programs more appropriately by supporting recovery efforts more specifically, reinforcing spiritual endeavors, making better referral decisions in regard to such programs, and making informed medication decisions.

The terminology requires a brief explanation. Due to the numerous Twelve Step programs and various conditions they address, the terms *addict* and *alcoholic* will be used interchangeably, with addict and addiction being a bit more prevalent. *Member* is used throughout the text to reference a participant in any Twelve Step program. The programs themselves can be very specific about their membership, but a working understanding of the principles of the Twelve Steps is the goal of this text.

It is the author's hope that the text will be of benefit to members of Twelve Step programs in at least two manners. The first is due to the basic premise of the text, that by establishment of an improved knowledge base, members will receive better care from clinicians. Second, members may directly benefit by reading the text for a fresh, thoughtful, perspective on the Steps.

1
Chapter One

A Practical Solution

Twelve Step programs have helped millions of people worldwide address addictive diseases of all types. These programs started in 1935 when Alcoholics Anonymous (A.A.) developed a practical program of action based on spiritual principles to help alcoholics abstain from drinking. The basis of the program is the Twelve Steps. These Steps, which have been described as a "design for living," have been altered for use by 73 different programs worldwide and are now used to help people who struggle with addictive or compulsive use of alcohol, narcotics, gambling, sex, and eating, among other problems.[1] These programs have grown rapidly since 1935, particularly in the past twenty years. For example, there are now more than 98,000 A.A. groups worldwide, with approximately 2 million people involved (see Table 1-1). It has been suggested that the Twelve Steps form the foundation of the most important and successful social movement of the twenty-first century. This is a bold statement to make about a spiritual program started by two desperate men in a last-ditch attempt to find relief from their own hopeless medical condition, alcoholism.

A medical school lecture about a disease that afflicts almost 20 percent (lifetime prevalence)[2] of people in the US and kills more than 200,000 people annually would likely attract a substantial audience. As the lecturer described how this pathology compared to other major medical illnesses—the third leading cause of preventable mortality in the US[3]—some in the audience would

TABLE 1-1. ESTIMATED A.A. MEMBERSHIP AND GROUP INFORMATION

Groups in US	51,183
Members in US	1,166,927
Groups in Canada	5,257
Members in Canada	101,786
Groups Overseas	39,804
Members Overseas	656,938
Internationalists	124
Groups in Correctional Facilities US/Canada	2,466
Lone Members	347
Total	
Members	1,989,124
Groups	98,710

begin to think about the incredible contributions they could make researching this dread disease. Unfortunately, once it was revealed that the topic was alcoholism and addiction, many in the audience would lose interest, and some would even argue that what was being discussed was not a disease at all. The lecturer could ask them to consider the large number of alcohol and drug related deaths, the morbidity and comorbid illness, but few would agree that this is one of the primary health problems in the US. Groups such as the American Society of Addiction Medicine (ASAM) have made remarkable inroads, but addictive disease remains largely outside the mainstream of medical education and research. While this has always been the case, there is evidence of progress. One can now find addictive disease on the curriculum of most medical schools in the US, and there has been a marked increase in the past ten years in the amount of research devoted to it, but it is certainly not given the time or money one would expect for an illness that affects such a large percentage of the population. Meanwhile, primary care physicians have to address the health problems directly and indirectly related to addiction on a daily basis; a review of the caseload of any hospital service will likewise reveal significant problems caused by chronic drug and alcohol abuse. Therapists are constantly presented with the problems of addicts and alcoholics and the family members of addicts and alcoholics. Yet it is estimated that only 15 percent of alcoholics receive the treatment they need. This is an illness that all health professionals face on a regular basis. Therefore, it is imperative that we have an understanding of Twelve Step programs, the most likely programs that people will use to address these diseases over their lifetime. The health professional with this knowledge will be in a position to provide appropriate treatment, care, and support to the numerous patients, family and friends that they encounter.

Twelve Step programs are considered mutual help or mutual support groups that emphasize abstinence from the addictive behavior. The individual members share their "experience, strength, and hope with one another."[4] They are not run by professionals, there are no group facilitators, and they have no supervision. Neither are Twelve Step programs treatment programs, though this is a common misconception and one that has actually been supported by some managed care programs. It is true that the principles of the Twelve Steps have been incorporated into many addiction treatment programs, and people often attend such meetings while in treatment programs. Furthermore, most addiction treatment programs will suggest that people attend Twelve Step meetings after treatment is completed, in order to develop a personal recovery program. Two factors recommend Twelve Step programs for this purpose: their accessibility and success. Both factors will be discussed later in this chapter. As changes in health care have resulted in increasingly limited access to treatment programs, individuals are in need of alternative means to address addiction problems. Twelve Step programs fill this void, as they did, in fact, before the development of modern treatment programs, when the addict had even fewer options. Prior to the founding of A.A., sanitariums and state hospitals had programs for inebriates, and sundry other "drying out" programs existed, but for the most part our culture was unaccepting of alcoholism and addictions. Certainly there was little consensus that addiction was a disease. As a result, only a limited few received any help at all. A.A. provided a safe haven, acceptance of the problem, and the help of dedicated members. In its infancy, only severe alcoholics would even consider such an attempt at addressing their problem; now addicts and alcoholics in varying stages of the disease use Twelve Step programs to alleviate suffering and arrest the disease process. And A.A. is now recognized throughout the world (Appendix 1, "Location of A.A. Groups or 'Loners'").

The Alcoholics Anonymous Preamble spells out the fundamental characteristics of Twelve Step programs:

> Alcoholics Anonymous is a fellowship of men and women who share their experience, strength and hope with each other that they may solve their common problem and help others to recover from alcoholism. The only requirement for membership is a desire to stop drinking. There are no dues or fees for A.A. membership; we are self-supporting through our own contributions. A.A. is not allied with any sect denomination, politics, organization or institution; does not wish to engage in any controversy; neither endorses nor opposes any causes. Our primary purpose is to stay sober and help other alcoholics to achieve sobriety.[5]

The Basic Characteristics of the Twelve Step Program.....

■ FELLOWSHIP

As the Alcoholics Anonymous Preamble states, A.A. is like a club, but one in which members develop a deep bond by revealing the tragedies of the disease and the triumphs found in recovery. Members share themselves at a level of intimacy surprising to the uninitiated. People often find themselves laughing at horrific life events with the knowledge that the others in the room have endured similar episodes and have forged ahead to reshape their lives based on the principles that bring them together. It is the devastation that brings these people together initially, but the hope they gain from others that keeps them coming back. People often refer to Twelve Step programs as self-help groups, but this is a mistake. These are mutual-help meetings, where people work together to meet common goals.

To become a member one needs only to attend a meeting and express interest in staying sober. "The only requirement for membership is a desire to stop drinking." There are no dues, no initiation fees, no assessment of need, and no evaluation. This is not treatment—one attends if one chooses to do so, without a gatekeeper. No one is required to do anything in a Twelve Step meeting. People attend and participate of their own free will, without bylaws or rules about expectations or conduct. Involvement is almost like joining a subculture with its own language, goals, and shared beliefs. The Twelve Steps are an approach to living, not just a means to alter an addictive behavior pattern. This is what attracts people; it constitutes the essence of the meetings and is the feature that brings people back: to join others in the exploration of self and the maintenance of abstinence. It is an experiential, verbal tradition of "one drunk talking to another" that cannot be fully understood without attending and witnessing the "miracle" of change that occurs in these peoples lives when they follow this spiritual path.

■ THE TWELVE STEP GROUP

The basic unit of activity in a Twelve Step program is the group. It is the core of the fellowship, governed in a very loose manner, providing the structure for the meetings themselves. The group can be considered administrative but functions more as an organizational body. In A.A. it is accepted that any time two or more alcoholics meet together for the purpose of maintaining sobriety they have established a group under the traditions of A.A. Most groups go beyond this minimalist definition to use officers and establish meeting procedures. The officers in any group are considered "trusted servants" and play important roles, but no officer or executive has authority over the group itself. A small group may use only a secretary–treasurer to provide necessary structure and handle finances. Volunteers regularly handle the housekeeping chores and refreshments. Larger groups may have numerous officers and a steering committee, including secretary, treasurer, chairperson, and general service representatives (GSR) who attend district or area meetings.

The group is also accountable for maintaining contact with the whole organization (see Figure 1-1). In A.A. this involves the GSR locally and at higher levels to represent themselves at the General Service Conference, an annual, international meeting where representatives share experience and hear reports from the General Service Board. The Board is composed of alcoholics and nonalcoholics who function as trustees and oversee A.A. World Services, Inc. and the A.A. Grapevine, Inc. The Board answers questions and addresses problems related to A.A. throughout the world. The Board also acts as custodian of the funds voluntarily contributed by groups to support the organization. There is a General Service Office in New York that serves as a clearinghouse for A.A. information and publications.* This is the best resource of A.A. literature. The General Service Board and the General Service Office consider themselves responsible to A.A. groups and have no authority over A.A. members or groups. This loosely structured democratic system functions under the traditions of A.A. as spelled out in the book *The Twelve Steps and Twelve Traditions* and respectfully attempts to make decisions based on the "consciousness" of A.A. as a whole.

As mentioned, each group is autonomous, able to hold any kind of meeting that it chooses, and functions with limited guidelines and recommendations. This allows for creative approaches, and the development of new groups to fit the needs of any particular community or sect. Acceptance of differences is emphasized in Twelve Step groups, but when needed, people can start their own particular type of group to address specific needs (see "Twelve Step Meetings," below). There is no cost or financial obligation associated with group involvement ("there are no dues or fees ..."). Groups will most often "pass the hat" during meetings ("we are self supporting through our own contributions ..."). This

---

* A.A. World Services, Inc., 475 Riverside Dr., 11th Floor, New York, NY 10115.

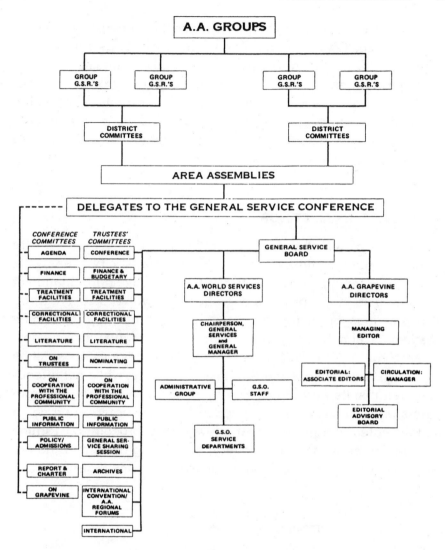

Figure 1-1 Structure of the Fellowship. *The A.A. Service Manual, 1979 Edition. Copyright 1969, A.A.*

money is used to pay rent, provide literature, provide refreshments, and to support the organization at higher levels. The group is simply responsible for keeping meetings dependable and effective, within the traditions of the Twelve Step program. No bylaws or rules about attendance, service work, or step work exist. One important function of the group is to make the community aware of its existence. One can find Twelve Step meetings through the local phone book, the newspaper, published meeting lists, and by asking a member. Outside of the meetings the group has other tasks, primarily associated with providing information or helping others directly through Twelve Step calls and working with local institutions. This includes providing information and volunteers to work with health care professionals.

■ TWELVE STEP MEETINGS

The main function of any group is to hold meetings. Meetings are available multiple times per day in any major city (see Table 1-2). The meetings provide a forum for the active participation of the members in the process of working a Twelve Step program. The meetings bring together people interested in maintaining abstinence and helping one another on a regular basis. Most research on A.A. as well as A.A. experience reveals, as shall be shown, that attendance tends to insure sobriety, while not attending often results in relapse. The meetings provide support from others who have had similar experiences. Newcomers are greeted and accepted in a manner that allows them to begin to examine themselves as worthy of recovery, something they often do not believe based on their behavior and the tragedies that may have

TABLE 1-2. PORTLAND, OREGON AREA
INTERGROUP A.A. MEETING DIRECTORY

	Number of meetings
Sunday	67
Monday	63
Tuesday	64
Wednesday	76
Thursday	62
Friday	65
Saturday	62
Daily	43
Monthly speaker meetings	7

resulted from their addictions. Most people arrive in a very desperate and needy state. The decision to attend meetings is not an easy one; most people consider it a last resort. Experienced members offer the newcomer the hope provided by their own experience in recovery. Education about the addictive process occurs, and a plan of recovery—"the way out"—begins to develop.

There are many types of meetings. Open meetings are for anyone interested in the Twelve Step program. They are open to the public, whether or not the attendee is there for his or her own recovery. Thus, a family member, friend, or even a health care worker may attend. Closed meetings are for the alcoholic or addict only. There are discussion meetings in which attendees will have the opportunity to talk. Speaker meetings have one or more speakers describing their own experience with the Twelve Steps; these are often open meetings. Meetings are now divided into smoking and nonsmoking meetings. Most meetings are not designated by gender, but men's and women's meetings exist. Specialty meetings are also available, offering people of a like mind or experience the opportunity to gather and share their own "experience, strength and hope" with each other, as it pertains to the Twelve Steps. These include meetings for African Americans and other ethnic groups, young people, gays, lesbians, doctors, lawyers, professionals, bikers, particular religious persuasions, newcomers, and even "old-timers." Specialty meetings will often ease the individual's initial trepidations with attending, and they are recommended for this purpose. Most A.A. old-timers will suggest such meetings be attended in addition to standard meetings which are more of a "melting pot" in order to allow the individual to more fully experience the "humanity" of these diseases. Meetings can be designated by the particular Twelve Step emphasis that occurs, such as Big Book meetings which study the A.A. text, Twelve Step meetings which focus specifically on the Steps, and Twelve Traditions meetings.

Discussion meetings are the most common. The group chairperson runs the meeting. The group usually opens with the serenity prayer ("God grant me the serenity to accept the things I cannot change, courage to change the things I can, and the wisdom to know the difference") followed by individual introductions, first name only, going around the room much like in a group therapy session, but limited to "My name is ____, and I'm an alcoholic" (or addict, chemically dependent, and so on according to how the individual chooses to identify him or herself). A particular reading may be used, such as the Preamble that is quoted above, the Twelve Steps, the Twelve Traditions, or another section of the *Alcoholics Anonymous* text (known as the "Big Book"), such as the first two and a half pages of chapter 5, "How It Works." The meeting secretary may give any Twelve Step related announcements. The "hat" is passed, with most people throwing in a dollar or two. The chairperson may introduce a topic with a short discussion, or a designated speaker will provide a "lead" commentary which is usually a discussion of a particular aspect of the Twelve Steps and how it pertains to that individual's recovery. Everyone in the room will be given an opportunity to speak, but they are not required to do so. The meetings last about an hour and usually end with another prayer. People tend to congregate before and after meetings, a more casual time to get to know each other and discuss their lives. It is not unusual for small groups of people to go out for coffee or other refreshments after the meeting. Friendships develop and more private conversations can take place.

There are no set rules or absolute recommendations about the number of meetings one should attend. Newcomers attend meetings more frequently than people that have been involved for longer periods. It is regularly suggested that people attend ninety meetings in ninety days when they enter a Twelve Step program without any formal treatment. When going through difficult life experiences, even members with longer term recovery will attend more frequently. The individual is always able to make the decision about this, but one can find patterns in different parts of the country. In major cities on the East and West coasts of the US, A.A. members tend to suggest daily meeting attendance. In the Midwest this is often not the case; members there often describe their meeting as a once a week affair. People choose a "home group" where they attend regularly and may involve themselves in organizational activities. This never limits them from attending other meetings.

■ WORKING A PROGRAM

"Working a program" is a phrase used by members of a Twelve Step group to describe their activities as they relate to recovery. John M. described this as "daily disciplines," the practices necessary to maintain sobriety and continue personal growth in recovery. Members recognize this as an individual program, and note that they are either growing and advancing in recovery or stagnant and retreating back toward the addictive behavior that got them there. Individuals must decide for themselves if a Twelve Step program is right for them. The meetings are available and they are helpful, but the addict needs to come to a position of acceptance of the disease and the need for help before he or she will attend these meetings and "work the program." The Twelve Steps are not theoretical but rather based on the experiences of early members of A.A. The steps reveal what these people found was necessary to maintain sobriety. If one is honestly ready to address the addiction, the Twelve Steps can provide a blueprint for recovery.

The list of activities involved in "working a program" is wide ranging and up to the individual, but behavioral in nature. Sometimes a sponsor or another member will recommend specific activities; sometimes members simply describe what they do on a daily and weekly basis to maintain their program. These practices can be readily examined, even measured, which can be a valuable self-assessment that can be used by the professional as well to come to an understanding of the Twelve Step member's progress. The most obvious activity is attending meetings. This is considered essential. Next in importance is "working the Steps"; that is, fully considering each of them in turn and actively engaging in the activity or alteration of thoughts and consciousness represented in the Step. Some of the Steps suggest activities that are incorporated into the daily lives of the member such as prayer, meditation, and a daily inventory (discussed in more detail later). Several daily meditation books are available to recovering addicts that are suggested as a way of starting the day off right, with a spiritual focus. (The first and most venerable of these type of books, written for recovering alcoholics, is *Twenty-four Hours a Day*.) Service work and volunteer activities are considered important aspects of an individual program. It is recommended that the Twelve Step member remain in contact with other members, whether by phone, computer or in person. Reading materials are available from the world service organizations of the various programs as well as other sources, and members suggest knowledge of the basic texts in each Twelve Step program (see Table 1-3)

Twelve Step programs are considered twenty-four hour a day programs. Thus, the individual is encouraged to decide to stay abstinent just for today. Newcomers often fixate on their disastrous pasts and how they will never be able to stay abstinent for the rest of their lives. The one-day-at-a-time emphasis of the Twelve Step program alleviates these concerns and places the focus on the only period one can do anything about, especially as it pertains to remaining sober: the present. The individual can stay sober *today*, can get to a meeting *today*, can contact someone *today*, and can work the steps *today*. A standard A.A. saying is, "Go to meetings and don't take the first drink."

Telling one's personal story is also included in working a program. Addiction is a disease marked by increasing isolation. The shame and guilt addicts carry often restricts their ability to connect with others. As the addiction worsens, denial becomes excessive and generalizes to prevent the individual from witnessing how drastically they have changed in most life spheres, not just in regard to the addictive behavior itself. Attending meetings with

TABLE 1-3. DAVE'S DAILY DISCIPLINES

- Upon waking, read *Twenty-four Hours a Day* and pray for ability to stay sober. Consider the day at hand
- Call my sponsor, contact another Twelve Step member
- Read from the Big Book
- Concentrate on one of the Steps
- Attend a meeting
- Complete a Tenth Step Inventory
- Prayer and meditation

others who understand this level of self-loathing, even self-hatred, can result in hope, and open the newcomer up in a manner which encourages the telling of their own tale. They witness others in good recovery who relate similar stories of the tragedy of addiction, then find themselves uplifted, and attracted to the possibility of a new way of life. In sharing themselves they begin the process of acceptance of this disease in a forum where others are already accepting of them. They find that in spite of their experiences they fit right in, that their stories help themselves and help others.

■ ABSTINENCE

Twelve Step programs recommend abstinence from the substance or behavior that is specific to the particular program. Thus A.A. recommends abstinence from alcohol, Narcotics Anonymous (N.A.) recommends abstinence from narcotics, and so on. The Twelve Steps do not specifically require abstinence—as mentioned, the only requirement for membership is a "desire to stop" using. Members understand, however, that the goal is abstinence. It should be noted that most people entering treatment programs have engaged in the use of more than one substance. The state of the art in addiction medicine is to recommend abstinence from all addicting, or mood altering, substances. There appears to be a final common pathway in addiction, and once a person has become addicted to one substance he or she is predisposed to addiction to any substance. The majority of people in Twelve Step programs understand this, and refrain from the use of all addicting substances, but again, it is not a requirement of any program. Those who do not take this seriously and want to continue to use a particular substance will use this loophole to justify ongoing drug or alcohol use. This will often occur with the cocaine addict who perceives alcohol has never been a problem. These people have missed an essential point about addictive disease, that the particular substance is of little importance. There are differences in the type of euphoric experience, the side effects, toxicity, and withdrawal, but in a general manner addiction runs a predictable course, independent of the substance. Thus the use of another substance that never resulted in addictive behavior has a predictable outcome: either addiction to the newly chosen "safe" substance or a quick return to addictive use of the prior drug of choice. Most members of Twelve Step programs understand this and incorporate it into their personal recovery program.

Advantages to the Clinician of Referring to Twelve Step Programs

■ ACCESSIBILITY

Anyone can attend Twelve Step programs. As mentioned, "the only requirement for membership is a desire to stop drinking" or using drugs or acting out sexually, and so on. Like all diseases, addiction can affect anyone, independent of nationality, profession, or social status. One can find Twelve Step meetings which exemplify a "melting pot" concept, with individuals who might otherwise never meet sharing a common bond forged through recovery. It is true that there are many different kinds of meetings and that one should be familiar with at least a few if referring individuals to Twelve Step recovery programs. A physician addict may not feel very comfortable at the local bikers meeting, and vice versa. Women now make up 34 percent of A.A. membership, making it easy to find dedicated female meetings.[*] A clinician should not hesitate, however, to refer anyone to a Twelve Step meeting. With a little effort, he or she can usually help find a meeting that particularly suits the client.

Health care has become extremely cost conscious. Addiction treatment has been cut back, like other treatments, to the barest essentials. This does not affect Twelve Step meetings, which are, as mentioned, self-supporting. The majority of meetings pass a hat into which people throw a dollar or two. Often it

---

[*] Alcoholics Anonymous 1998 Membership Survey, A.A. World Services.

is suggested that the newcomer should not even contribute. Most programs will have a listed phone number, and one can contact them for a ride to and from the meetings. This would not result in a fee, most members consider this "service work," and it is gladly offered.

There are large Twelve Step meeting networks in most major cities. These organizations are usually published in the white pages, and are very easy to access. (This is not necessarily true for Sex Addicts Anonymous, and similar meetings, which may require a personal contact to locate.) Published meeting lists are available which provide meeting times and places. These can be handed out to people, or made available in your office. It is fair to state that A.A. meetings are occurring multiple times daily in any major city. The meetings are often found in churches or community centers. A.A. club houses exist that provide space for meetings on a daily basis. These clubs also often offer social activities for people in recovery. They can be accessed through the local intergroup or central office, which will have a phone number in the local directory. In addition to formal resources, people are actually available twenty-four hours a day. These organizations will provide a contact for newcomers or for an interested health care worker.

A.A. meetings and many of the other Twelve Step meetings are available worldwide. The A.A. Central Service Office publishes a directory of meetings around the world. Many people enjoy attending such meetings overseas. A.A. literature is published in 41 languages. The meeting format is roughly the same independent of the country or language, and these meetings can be a lifesaver for the world traveler who needs support. The World Wide Web also has numerous sites for Twelve Step meetings and chat rooms (see Appendix 2, "Twelve Steps on the World Wide Web"). This allows people to access meetings at any time and provides a means of support for those unable to get away to a meeting.

■ **A TRADITION OF CARING: SERVICE WORK**

"Service work" is emphasized in Twelve Step programs. This includes various voluntary efforts that help the program or the individual. Because Twelve Step programs emphasize helping others, they represent an extraordinary resource for the health care worker. Members are willing to be called upon by their peers when help is needed. It is not unusual for an A.A. or N.A. member to tell someone to call any time of day or night if needed to help address a problem related directly or indirectly to maintaining sobriety. This is not advertised or described, it is a given. Twelve Step members will go out of their way for one another, and refer to it as "Twelfth Step work." A.A. was founded on an understanding that the individual can keep sobriety only by giving it away. Twelve Step members' efforts on behalf of one another result from this belief. Most members view this as giving back what was so freely given to them when they were newcomers.

One aspect of service work is "sponsorship." People in Twelve Step programs pick a sponsor to talk to outside of the meetings for a more in-depth understanding of the program. Sponsors are usually of the same sex as the individual, have more experience in the program (at least a year), and are willing to provide direction and teach others about their own understanding of "working the Steps." Sponsors become confidantes, provide advice, and indoctrinate the newcomer into practical applications of the Twelve Steps. The relationship is not unlike that of a student with a teacher, but the sponsor can be considered a sounding board, a guide, a role model, and a mentor. An expectation for honest disclosure is presumed, and people share themselves at an intimate level. Sponsor/sponsee relationships often evolve into lifelong friendships. Groups recommend that members each have a sponsor, especially the newcomer. Newcomers have myriad questions and problems as they begin to attend meetings, and these can often be immediately addressed by a sponsor. A sponsor will provide direction in regard to specific aspects of the individual Steps and may even suggest reading, workbook, or other assignments. People use their sponsors for any life issues that come up, whether they seem to be A.A. related or not.

Service work involves wide ranging activities. A popular one is making coffee for others at the meeting site. Someone has to open the building or the room, set up the chairs, and clean up after meetings. Each group has a secretary and a treasurer. As mentioned, volunteers answer phones and help others with rides to and from meetings. Members volunteer as speakers at meetings and for community organizations. "When anyone anywhere, reaches out for help, I want the hand of A.A. always to be there. And for that: I am responsible."*

Twelfth Step work, also called a Twelfth Step call, is considered an essential service. This is an activity emphasized in Step Twelve: "Having had a spiritual awakening as a result of these steps, we tried to carry this message to alcoholics ..." A.A. members often refer to the first meeting of the cofounders, Dr. Bob Smith and Bill Wilson, as the first Twelfth Step call. Twelve Step groups are often contacted by people in need of help. A Twelfth Step call may involve members visiting with someone who is still in active addiction. It is recommended that at least two members go on such visits. The members share their "experience, strength and hope," essentially describing their own addiction and recovery: "what we used to be like, what happened, and what we are like now."[6] Many people enter Twelve Step programs in this manner, or enter into formal treatment programs as a result of these efforts. Often members talk with addicts while the addicts are intoxicated, and it can be dangerous. In the past, when treatment was unavailable, members would help in detoxing others. This is seldom necessary anymore, but the practice still exists, especially in areas with limited treatment resources. It is important to note that a Twelfth Step call is considered successful when the *members* come away from it sober; success is not gauged by the effect on the active addict. This is because the emphasis is on sharing the program to maintain one's own sobriety, not to elicit it in others.

Members of A.A. are regularly approached by health care workers with questions and requests for help. The A.A. members take this seriously, and groups even have committees devoted to liaison with health care workers and the community, the

---

* A.A. World Services.

Committees on Cooperation with the Professional Community. These committees are found in any major city and usually serve large areas with the intent of informing professionals about what A.A. can and cannot do. They can also be a resource for information on alcoholism and addiction treatment services in the area. A.A. publishes a pamphlet for clinicians, "For the Professional," which is available through the local A.A. club or the General Service office in New York. Twelve Step program members have the ability to provide information about addiction based on their own experience, which is a powerful message unique to them. Their literature readily admits that they do not help others based on scientific or professional expertise. Their message is one of firsthand knowledge of the problem and a solution based on the Twelve Steps. Thus they can work with the professional, and provide a realistic, practical, approach to helping the active addict/alcoholic. Most people in the midst of these diseases are very sensitive to criticism, and often complain that health care workers blame them, and even berate them. These people are experiencing tremendous inner pain and conflict, have beat themselves up, are ashamed of their behavior, guilt ridden, and often feel hopeless, yet cannot determine how to change. Condescension or blame from an authority figure are often more than they can bear. A Twelve Step member on a Twelfth Step call is sharing a common experience, however, at a level of understanding only gained through intimate knowledge of the same pain, and can reach out to the suffering with a message of hope and the ultimate example of their own sobriety. This is a powerful tool that can be readily accessed by a health care worker with a call to a Twelve Step program.

■ PERSONAL RESPONSIBILITY

Twelve Step programs make a point of placing responsibility for the problem right where it belongs, with the addicts/alcoholics themselves. The alcoholic/addict is expected within a Twelve Step program to be accountable for his or her past behavior, for the addiction, and for recovery. This is confounding to the observer due to our views of other diseases as well as legal opinions about responsibility.* We have a tendency to think that illness implies that responsibility is relinquished, and this is not the case. Ask any diabetic who is ultimately responsible for their blood sugar, their diet and their insulin. The addict/alcoholic must attend to the basics of a recovery program that works; attend meetings, share themselves with others, and work the Steps. Without doing so, relapse is inevitable. Twelve Step programs are voluntary, and the individual only attends if they have a "desire to stop" using. The individual is responsible for attending meetings and for working a personal recovery program, if they choose to, without anyone else in control of the effort or the outcome. The individual is also accountable for his or her own behavior—no one is caring for the addict, although peers will offer support and guidance. Some argue that considering addiction a disease abdicates all responsibility for the behavior that occurs during active addiction, such as DWIs or violent acts committed under the influence of a psychoactive substance. Twelve Step programs do not consider this legitimate; in fact, Twelve Step programs direct the addict/alcoholic to account for past transgressions and to make amends for them.

Addiction is not a disease that can be cured. The health care worker is not responsible for a cure, nor can the addict expect a cure that would allow a return to recreational or social use. Health care workers must recognize that they play an important role in helping the addict retain sobriety, but that the role is limited. Responsibility for ongoing recovery, for abstinence, is up to the individual. Twelve Step programs recognize and emphasize this.

■ DO TWELVE STEP PROGRAMS WORK?

A.A. meetings often end with the phrase "keep coming back, it works." The success of Twelve Step programs is indicated in the number of members, but is supported by only limited research. A.A. has spawned numerous Twelve Step recovery

---

* It should be noted that these programs do not define the problem, nor do they refer to it as disease. They leave this to the professionals.

programs to address other addictive behaviors. A.A. is now found in over 170 countries and boasts over 2 million members. Research on Twelve Step programs is limited due to the nature of the programs and specific boundaries set by their governing bodies. George E. Vaillant, in his text *The Natural History of Alcoholism*, states, "Alcoholism is a problem that affects millions of people. The development of a treatment that does not spread in exponential fashion (as have for example, penicillin, Alcoholics Anonymous, and renal dialysis) cannot be regarded as particularly helpful."[7] A.A. has spread, and is considered the most effective community-based therapy for alcoholism. Once again, A.A. is not treatment, but describes itself as a worldwide fellowship in which people can participate if they want to remain abstinent from alcohol.

The results of a 1998 A.A. survey of 6,800 A.A. members from the US and Canada revealed more about the success of A.A. Sixty-six percent of the membership were male, and 34 percent female, a ratio of approximately 2:1. In the under-thirty age group, 62 percent were male and 38 percent female. These numbers suggest an over-representation of women, since it was determined by the Epidemiologic Catchment Area studies that the ratio of men to women with an alcohol abuse/dependence disorder in the prior month in a community sample was approximately 5:1.[8] The A.A. survey also revealed that the average length of sobriety was greater than seven years, with 27 percent under one year, 26 percent between one and five years, and 47 percent over five years. The four most likely factors leading to A.A. involvement were: brought in by an an A.A. member, 36 percent; referred by a treatment facility, 34 percent; self-referred, 34 percent; and referred by family, 25 percent. The percentage referred by a health care provider was surprisingly low at 8 percent. In spite of the growth and success of A.A., health care professionals continue to neglect this important tool in the care of alcoholics.[*]

---

[*] Alcoholics Anonymous 1998 Membership Survey, A.A. World Services.

As mentioned, research on Twelve Step programs is lacking due in part to numerous barriers inherent to the programs. Nonetheless, A.A. does support research endeavors, though the organization is clear that its program addresses the alcoholic and leaves alcoholism to the scientists. From their perspective, Twelve Step programs are successful and well established; many people have a great deal of confidence in them. This results in little organizational interest in scientific examination, as change is not considered necessary. These programs are not based on a medical model, they are not treatment programs, and they have stood the test of time. The A.A. traditions state that "A.A. is not allied with any sect, denomination, politics, organization, or institution."[9] This can present a problem for research by any particular organization. Each group is autonomous, receiving only limited guidance for general activities; thus, meetings are remarkably variable, which undermines attempts at scientific inquiry. Because meetings are set up solely for the sobriety of the members and anonymity is strictly adhered to, research activities must be done outside of the actual meetings. Furthermore, as shall be discussed in the next chapter, the foundation of a Twelve Step program is spiritual, something very difficult to measure and quantify. These programs will not be altered to assist in research, but A.A. suggests that individuals involve themselves in such research whenever appropriate. Bill Wilson, an A.A. cofounder, wrote, "Today the vast majority of us welcome any new light that can be thrown on the alcoholic's mysterious and baffling malady. We welcome new and valuable knowledge, whether it issues from a test tube, from a psychiatrist's couch or from revealing social studies."[*]

The bulk of the research that has been done on Twelve Step programs has been done with A.A., and it addresses two primary issues: the characteristics of the participants and abstinence as it relates to participation. Emrich wrote that demographic variables including education, sex, age, and marital status had little correla-

---

[*] Alcoholics Anonymous World Services memo on participation of A.A. members in research and other non-A.A. surveys.

tion with Twelve Step fellowship participation.[10] In a different study he found no specific A.A. personality, and noted that more severe alcoholics were more likely to attend.[11] Thurston, Alfano, and Sherer used pretreatment MMPI profiles of A.A. members and nonmembers to examine personality differences among those attending A.A. regularly and those who did not. As they found no personality differences, A.A. attendance was not noted to be pre-dictable based on personality traits.[12] Many therapists are un-aware of this finding. A common (unfortunate) explanation for avoiding referral to Twelve Step programs is that the client has inappropriate personality traits.

In *Principles of Addiction Medicine*, Dupont and Shiraki state, "The two central research findings from longitudinal studies of alcoholics and drug addicts are that: (1) Although many alcoholics and drug addicts become abstinent without attending Twelve Step meetings, most studies show that a large percentage of long-term recovering alcoholics and addicted persons attribute their success to Twelve Step meeting attendance; and (2) long-term and fre-quent Twelve Step meeting attendance correlates positively with long-term abstinence from the use of alcohol and other drugs."[13] Vaillant found that the individuals who derived the most benefit from A.A. attended an average of 300 meetings in the eight-year follow-up period. He also noted that alcoholics who became absti-nent through A.A. varied greatly in their attendance and level of involvement.[14]

Multiple research studies have shown a positive correlation between A.A. attendance and abstinence. Thurston, Alfano, and Nerviano revealed that half of the patients treated in an inpatient setting remained abstinent at eighteen months after treatment.[15] Emrick described a positive correlation between A.A. participa-tion before and after addiction treatment with long-term absti-nence from alcohol. He also noted several aspects of A.A. participation that correlated with positive outcomes: having a sponsor, participating in A.A. activities, conducting meetings, and increasing ones involvement in a Twelve Step group.[16] Sheeren found that active involvement in A.A. reduced relapse rate.[17] Galanter et al. (1990) studied 100 impaired physicians who described A.A. as the primary element contributing to their recovery.[18]

A.A. attendance appears to correlate with abstinence from alcohol, and active A.A. participation is described as having a positive correlation on long-term abstinence. These two facts, established in research, are well known to the members of Twelve Step groups. There also appears to be no frank evidence of an alcoholic personality, nor can researchers determine a type of personality that will do best in A.A.; thus clinicians should not rule out A.A. as a source of support for recovery from alcoholism based on bias about an individual's personality or Twelve Step groups. Twelve Step groups have grown dramatically because they work. The ability for A.A. to establish meetings in countries outside the US, and in vastly different cultures suggests that its success is not limited to a certain subculture. From an academic perspective, more research on the efficacy of the Twelve Steps is needed. Though these programs are not in the treatment business, they are in the business of helping alcoholics and addicts help each other recover from alcoholism and addictions, and they therefore support attempts to further the understanding of the disease.

■ REFERRING TO MEETINGS

For the health care professional it is good to have a routine in referring people to Twelve Step programs. Research by Sisson and Mallams (1981) helps to understand the need for established contacts in Twelve Step groups. They randomly assigned newly diagnosed alcoholics to two groups and referred them to A.A. One group was told to call A.A. on their own and attend a meeting. None of them attended. The second group was provided direct contact with an A.A. member by a phone call from the physician's office. All members of the second group attended an A.A. meeting.[19] This reveals the importance of Twelve Step contacts that can provide this type of service, and the usefulness of a list of people to call upon. It should also be noted that most groups emphasize the type of service work that results in a willingness to help the health professional in these circumstances. Health care workers can obtain a list of meetings from the local office of A.A. or N.A. The lists will describe the time, place, and type of meeting. These lists will also usually provide contacts or a phone number to gain more information. As mentioned, most major cities also have large "clubs" that offer twenty-four hour information services.

REFERENCES

1. Barbara J. White and Edward J. Madara, comp. and ed., *The Self-Help Sourcebook: Finding and Forming Mutual Aid Self-Help Groups, 5th Ed.* (Denville, NJ: American Self-Help Clearinghouse, 1995).
2. D. A. Regier et al., Co-morbidity of mental disorders with alcohol and other drug abuse: Results of the environmental catchment area study, *JAMA*, 1990, 264(19): 2511–2518.
3. (Alcohol only) Actual causes of death in the United States, *JAMA*, 1993, 270(18): 2208.
4. *Alcoholics Anonymous Preamble*, A.A. Grapevine, 1947.
5. *Ibid.*
6. *Alcoholics Anonymous* (New York: A.A. World Services, Inc., 1976) p. 58.
7. George E. Vaillant, *The Natural History of Alcoholism* (Cambridge, MA: Harvard University Press, 1983) p. 234.
8. J.E. Helzer, A. Burnam, and L.T. McElroy, Alcohol abuse and dependence, in: L.N. Robins and D.A. Regier, eds., *Psychiatric Disorders in America: The Epidemiologic Catchment Area Study* (New York: The Free Press, 1991) pp. 81–115.
9. *Alcoholics Anonymous Preamble*, A.A. Grapevine, 1947.
10. C.D. Emrich, Alcoholics Anonymous and other 12-Step groups: Establishing an empirically based approach for the health care provider, in: M. Galanter, ed., *The Treatment of Substance Abuse* (Washington, DC: American Psychiatric Press, 1994).
11. C.D. Emrich, Alcoholics Anonymous: Affiliation processes and effectiveness as treatment, *Brown University Digest of Addiction Theory and Application*, 1988, 7: 66–69.

12. A.H. Thurston, A.M. Alfano, and M. Sherer, Pretreatment MMPI profiles of A.A. members and nonmembers, *Journal of Alcohol Studies*, 1986, 47:468–471.
13. R. L. Dupont and S. Shiraki, Twelve Step programs, in: Norman Miller, ed., *Principles of Addiction Medicine*, Chapter 5 (Chevy Chase, MD: American Society of Addiction Medicine, 1994).
14. George E. Vaillant, *The Natural History of Alcoholism* (Cambridge, MA: Harvard University Press, 1983).
15. A.H. Thurston, A.M. Alfano, and V.J. Nerviano, The efficacy of A.A. attendance for aftercare of inpatient alcoholics: Some follow-up data, *International Journal of the Addictions*, 1987, 22:1083–1090.
16. C.D. Emrich, J.S. Tonigen, H. Montgomery, and L. Little, Alcoholics Anonymous: What is currently known? in: B.S. McGrady and W.R. Miller, eds., *Research on A.A.: Opportunities and Alternatives* (Brunswick, NJ: Rutgers Center for Alcohol Studies, 1993).
17. M. Shereen, The relationship between relapse and involvement in Alcoholics Anonymous, *Journal of Studies on Alcohol*, 1988, 49: 104–106.
18. M. Galanter, D. Talbott, K. Gallegos, and E. Robenstone, Combined A.A. and professional care for addicted physicians, *American Journal of Psychiatry*, 1990, 147: 64–68.
19. R.W. Sisson and J.H. Mallams, The use of systematic encouragement and community access procedures to increase attendance at Alcoholics Anonymous and Al-Anon meetings, *American Journal of Drug Abuse*, 1981, 8(3): 371–376.

2

Chapter Two

Spiritual Experience

Appendix II, "Spiritual Experience," of *Alcoholics Anonymous* ends with the following quote by Herbert Spencer: "There is a principle which is a bar against all information, which is proof against all arguments and which cannot fail to keep a man in everlasting ignorance—that principle is contempt prior to investigation." This quote is used here as an opening statement to orient us to the foundation of any Twelve Step program, spirituality. No apologies are made, and it is a frank emphasis. This emphasis can bewilder the newcomer and the clinician. Yet, it is believed that the solution to addiction and alcoholism lies in spiritual discipline. "The spiritual life is not a theory. We have to live it."[1] This chapter attempts to provide an understanding of what this means to the members of Twelve Step programs and provide the clinician with comprehension of some of the spiritual principles used in these programs. *Alcoholics Anonymous* puts it this way:

> The great fact is just this, and nothing less: That we have had deep and effective spiritual experiences which have revolutionized our whole attitude toward life, toward our fellows and toward God's universe. The central fact of our lives today is the absolute certainty that our Creator has entered into our hearts and lives in a way which is indeed miraculous. He has commenced to accomplish those things for us which we could never do by ourselves.[2]

Twelve Step programs are based on the experience of people who, out of desperation, began to examine their lives based on spiritual principles. This spiritual influence preceded the establishment of the program itself as found on this brief description of the first meeting of the cofounders of A.A., Bill Wilson and Dr. Robert Smith. From the very beginning there was a resistance to formal religion, and, over time, an emphasis on the distinction between religion and spirituality. Wilson and Smith met in 1935, a time when alcoholism was considered by medical professionals to be a hopeless condition. Bill W. had been making unsuccessful attempts to quit drinking, using most of the available methods, when he had a sudden, dramatic, "spiritual experience." This event was inspired by an alcoholic friend, Ebby T., who had a conversion experience with the Oxford Group, a nondenominational, conservative, Christian, evangelical, movement. Ebby T. had visited Bill W. to explain to a fellow alcoholic about his newfound cure. Bill found it very disturbing when told by Ebby, "I've got religion." Wilson was suspicious and initially assumed that Ebby, who he had viewed as a hopeless drunk, was now going to preach to him. This was, however, the beginning of "one alcoholic talking to another" as Ebby did not preach to Bill but merely discussed with him their common plight. Bill's "spiritual experience" occurred at the end of his last binge, while hospitalized under the care of Dr. William Silkworth. After the hospitalization Bill involved himself in the Oxford Group, examined their principles, and set out to help other alcoholics. He began to realize the special needs of alcoholics as he worked with many who were unable to remain abstinent.

Bill W. went to Akron, Ohio, in May 1935, on business, and while there began to consider drinking. He desperately sought out another alcoholic to talk to, with the idea that only this would keep him from using alcohol again. Through an Oxford Group connection he met Dr. Bob. A.A. considers this meeting the founding moment of the A.A. fellowship and therefore the founding of Twelve Step programs. Dr. Bob's involvement in the Oxford Group was already established and the two of them immersed themselves in its teachings and practice. They supported each other for a period of several months and enrolled others into their way of thinking about abstinence. They separated when Bill returned to New York and established a group there. As the movement grew, so did the recognition that the Oxford Group was too religious for many of the people with whom they were working. Wilson, Smith, and other founding members realized that they needed to specifically distinguish spirituality from religion, allowing anyone access to their method of abstinence. They attempted to walk a fine line with this approach, one that did not alienate those of a particular religious persuasion yet allowed for those who would reject religious teachings. Their efforts resulted in a method to help alcoholics, based on spiritual principles, that was inclusive and balanced the nonreligious with the religious within their midst, establishing a middle ground based on the individual's interpretation and understanding of a "higher power." They allied with no particular religion yet gained acceptance of their mission from a wide variety of religious traditions.

In *Not-God: A History of Alcoholics Anonymous*, Ernest Kurtz addressed the events that established the A.A. program as well as the significance of A.A. in the history of religious thought. " 'Not God' means first 'You are not God,' the message of the A.A. program. ... The fundamental and first message of Alcoholics Anonymous to its members is that they are not infinite, not absolute, *not God.* ... But Alcoholics Anonymous is fellowship as well as program, and thus there is a second side to its message of not-God-ness. Because the alcoholic is not God, not absolute, not infinite, he or she is essentially limited. Yet from this very limitation—from the alcoholic's acceptance of personal limitation—arises the beginning of healing and wholeness."[3] These thoughts reveal the deeply religious nature of A.A. principles, which are established in a Twelve Step program as spiritual, thus open to the interpretation of the individual, and inclusive by their very nature. Kurtz points out that "the acceptance of the philosophy of pluralism such as A.A.'s—the capacity to accept difference as enriching rather than threatening and the ability to flourish within the context of the shared honesty of mutual vulnerability openly acknowledged—requires that the *basis of sharing be weakness rather than strength*. That strength arises precisely from weakness is the ancient and first fundamental religious insight. It is also precisely the insight to which among myriad of phenomena that dot the historical landscape of America in the twentieth century, Alcoholics Anonymous best, if not also alone, witnesses with a clarity and simplicity that render its wisdom readily, easily, and vividly understandable by all and accessible to all.[4] Strength flows from the recognition of limitation—alcoholism or addiction—resulting in the ability to turn to a power outside oneself. Active alcoholics continue to drink without recognition of this limitation; their illness is enveloped in denial. Acceptance of limitation can open one to the humanity of one's situation: not-God, but finite human. The early members, beaten into submission by alcohol, had little recourse, and recognized spiritual discipline as a way out. In attempting to develop a spiritual program that would not be rejected by the very people that they set out to help, the founders emphasized a simple program of action that developed into the Twelve Steps. They described the alcoholic, not alcoholism, recognizing another limitation of their own understanding and basing their program on experience. Spiritual principles based on limitation were the basis for their sobriety, their growth, and their very lives. "We are not cured of alcoholism. What we really have is a daily reprieve contingent on the maintenance of our spiritual condition."[5]

Many health care professionals actually face the same quandary as the newcomer to a Twelve Step program: how can I believe this? The spiritual emphasis includes using prayer to open and close meetings; the word God is found in the literature; and open discussions of spiritual beliefs are commonplace. This immediately reveals biases and, often, strong responses, both positive and negative. The founders attempted to eliminate these problems as much as possible, but by nature it is controversial. People find themselves influenced by their religious upbringing, their religious preferences, and even their professional training as they scrutinize the spirituality of the Twelve Steps. There are distinct Christian overtones, and this can immediately pose problems for those of other religious orientations, as well as for the agnostic and atheist.

Questions about cults and religious fanatics arise. At first glance these programs seem anything but the inclusive, open programs they proclaim to be. Some people immediately reject them without looking beyond their initial response.

The clinician may be faced with other questions. There is no training in spiritual perspectives for most medical and mental health professionals, in spite of evidence that people rank their religious and spiritual beliefs to be essential to their very existence. Fortunately this is changing as training programs are examining nontraditional approaches, and more therapists are making the spiritual an emphasis. Nonetheless, some professionals believe discussion of the spiritual to be unprofessional; some adhere to Freud's view that such beliefs are a form of neurosis; and some even suggest that addressing the spiritual concerns of clients is worthless or perhaps even damaging. A major argument is the lack of scientific data giving credence to the idea of spiritual healing, but this is changing. Larry Dossey, M.D. has substantiated a significant body of literature devoted to the examination of healing through spiritual and religious means.

Such professional biases need to be addressed in order to successfully work with the client who chooses or is referred to a Twelve Step program. The addict is often acting out of desperation, and hopelessness, while the clinician is objectively examining treatment strategies. The addict may be in a life-threatening situation, as the clinician considers therapeutic options. The addict is taught to take responsibility for his or her own recovery in a Twelve Step program, while the health care professional is often trained in such a manner that they believe they must be responsible for the client. As mentioned, Twelve Step programs are mutual help programs and have no supervision. This can be unsettling to the professional. In addition, the addict may only tell the professional part of their history, which can compromise therapeutic goals. While this can also happen in a Twelve Step meeting, due to the level of honest sharing in these groups it is very likely that a person will begin to open up as modeled by other members and without the same degree of guilt and shame that can pervade the therapeutic relationship. The spiritual emphasis of the Twelve

Step meetings can begin to help the active addict move from the helplessness and hopelessness of addiction to a sense of reawakening of the human spirit. This is the beginning of hope, which can result in dramatic life change if the individual is able to live using the spiritual tools presented in the Twelve Steps. In this manner the new member begins to "live the program."

In examining the Twelve Steps one finds a distinct emphasis on the individual's conception of God. References to God are vague and left to personal interpretation: "a Power greater than ourselves" and "God as we understood Him." This empowers the individual to examine his or her own ideas about a higher power in an attempt to eliminate as much religious bias as possible. The result is an inclusive forum from which people can safely build a fundamental understanding of spiritual discipline based on active participation in a simple program.

When the early members of A.A. broke from the Oxford Group they recognized that an inclusive stance was necessary to maintain an alcoholic's involvement in a program that had a spiritual emphasis. They did not specifically define this form of spirituality and one cannot find a definition in the Twelve Step literature. Thus, the individual must develop a working definition based on their life experience and the support of their peers in Twelve Step meetings. No member will even begin to define for another what "God as we understood Him" means. "When, therefore, we speak to you of God, we mean your conception of God. This applies, too, to other spiritual expressions which you find in this book. Do not let any prejudice you may have against spiritual terms deter you from honestly asking yourself what they mean to you."[6] Still, for some it is difficult to address anything spiritual. They cringe as they begin the process of facing the language used in the meetings and the literature. Others are confused by the emphasis on an individual approach allowing for one's own definition. The professional can aid in this search for meaning, but only with an understanding of these principles. Otherwise, the clinician can contribute to the problems and confusion. Conversely, the clinician who understands the Twelve Steps can use them as an adjunct to therapeutic approaches, for the Twelve Steps address common human conditions with a spiritual approach that is simple, uses direct principles, and is readily understandable. The spiritual solution is described as a "design for living" which results in more than just abstinence from addictive behavior, but a better life grounded in the perennial philosophies.

Just as the participant in a Twelve Step program has no frank definition of spirituality to use as a guide, the professional is left to examine spirituality for themselves and their clients as well. It bears repeating that the health care professional has the opportunity to be of tremendous service in helping the individual come to an understanding of these spiritual concepts. A thorough understanding of the principles of Twelve Step spirituality is necessary for the professional to work in a productive manner that enhances the individual's spiritual program rather than detracting from it. The professional must come to recognize and honor "God as we understood Him" in a manner that can be communicated to the individual just as inclusively as it would be in a Twelve Step meeting. Since Twelve Step groups endorse other spiritual and religious disciplines and activities, the professional open to and aware of the level of inclusiveness in this construct can use their own varied backgrounds to understand these concepts and work with clients. Using a spiritual approach rather than a religious one also eliminates a level of dogma that can be a pitfall when addressing people in Twelve Step programs. One has to steadfastly avoid preaching, yet be able to communicate a solid understanding of spiritual principles, especially how the Twelve Steps are considered an active practice of spiritual principle, not a theological argument. This level of understanding and openness to this way of thinking is very well received by clients in Twelve Step programs and fosters improvement in the therapeutic relationship.

The professional can also use an understanding of the spiritual aspects of a Twelve Step program as an assessment tool, much like people within these programs do for each other. A general examination of the individual's understanding of spirituality will give one information pertinent to their level of involvement in a recovery program. Most active Twelve Step members can readily describe spiritual disciplines and activities that have enhanced their lives and will do so using language specific to a Twelve Step program with examples from the Steps themselves that emphasize their own conception of God. This will reveal the level of involvement in the specific steps and their understanding of these Steps. This form of evaluation can actually be of benefit in assessing risk for relapse or other maladaptive behaviors. Lacking a definition of spirituality, one must use knowledge of these principles, in communication, rather than a specific set of criteria.

The story is told of a physician who was an atheist when he entered A.A. He took the individual's conception of a higher power to the extreme. His initial involvement in A.A. was somewhat frustrating for him due to the spiritual emphasis. He became willing to try out the A.A. way when he considered the success that others had with it, since all his efforts had failed to result in abstinence. Ultimately he was faced with choosing a higher power, and chose a doorknob. He said it was outside himself, he had no control over it, and the metaphor of opening doors for him was appealing. It sounds unusual, and one can question the effectiveness of such an approach, but it worked for him. He understood it as a power outside himself, which he turned to for help. However, his concept of a higher power shifted over time. He began to recognize some of the limitations of the doorknob metaphor as higher power, and chose his group instead. This also worked for a period of time. He maintained that the group was clearly a power greater than himself, and he trusted them to hold his best interest at heart. Ultimately he began to discuss a higher power that was not of this material world. Although he used different concepts of a higher power, they all served the same general purpose, as he recognized that he was "not God" and that he required an outside influence to work the spiritual aspects of a Twelve Step program. His experience is also in keeping with the majority of people who enter Twelve Step programs. Appendix II of *Alcoholics Anonymous* describes this phenomenon: "Most of our experiences are what the psychologist William James calls the 'educational variety' because they develop slowly over a period of time."

Just as there are many forms of "God as we understood Him," there are many ways of referring to God in a Twelve Step program. God may be the most common, and some point out that it is a single syllable, easy to say, and people have a general idea what one is referring to when they use this term. Some use god as an acronym for "good orderly direction." Higher Power, or HP, is also very commonly used. Almost anything goes, as people use Great Spirit, the force, benevolent one, mother earth, etc. This can be difficult for some people with fairly traditional Christian views, as they may be rigid about the use of the word God and its meaning. The result may be an inability to get involved in a Twelve Step program. All of this speaks to the inclusive nature of these programs, an emphasis that is imperfect, but tends to limit problems with a spiritual approach.

In talking with members of Twelve Step groups, I found no evidence of a definition or specific strategy to use in coming to understand the spirituality of these programs. They all stated that it is up to the individual to decide for him or herself what a spiritual awakening means. Some call it an act of surrender and an act of humility because it reveals our human limits and the requirement for help in addressing this life-threatening illness. Some reference the selfish nature of this illness, something they all recognized during their active addictions but could do nothing about until they began to examine their lives from a spiritual perspective and concluded, "I'm not the center of the universe." Again, it cannot be defined by anyone for anyone else but only recognized as the individual experiences it. Members often claim simply that they know it when they experience it and when they see it in others.

To convey what it may be like to experience the incredible relief as well as the unleashing of human potential that comes with successfully addressing an addiction by relying on a higher power, Cheryl M. suggested examination of the extraordinary aspects of daily life: What elicits awe and wonder? What leaves when we die? Where does love come from? What inspires you? What does it mean to feel connected with someone? How do we have an inner sense of right and wrong? Where does an original thought come from? What does it mean to be alive? For the recovering addict, and perhaps for anyone, once awareness of the human spirit is experienced the individual can begin to evolve. This evolution can manifest in a multitude of ways. In a Twelve Step program it is founded on a simple program of action outlined in the Steps, but the paths are many and varied. The "joke" for many newcomers is that one does not just stop using, one has to change one's whole life. These changes are the true gift of a spiritual path and why the Twelve Steps are not just about abstinence but also about the opportunity for life change and growth.

In talking with recovering people it becomes clear that they use many other methods of addressing themselves in a spiritual manner. Most do not limit their understanding nor their spiritual activities to the Twelve Steps. Prayer and meditation are suggested in the Steps, and most members use these disciplines. Some attend church regularly and practice the forms and rituals of a specific religion. Many regularly read about spirituality from a variety of resources, revealing an acceptance of multiple religious perspectives. Some have worked A Course in Miracles or followed a specific spiritual teacher. Twelve Step members attend conferences and retreats to enhance their understanding of their spiritual selves. It is evident in their activities that spirituality becomes a major focus in their lives.

One member described an attraction to discussions of spirituality upon entering A.A. He had grown up Lutheran but no longer attended church. Yet he longed for a sense of meaning in his life. His addiction had taken away any shred of belief that God may exist and left him with mountains of guilt and shame regarding his behavior. In the examples of the older members he began to glimpse hope, however, that perhaps he could be like them—if they could do it, he may have a chance as well. Old-timers spoke of God, of a Higher Power, and of turning their lives over. They seemed genuinely happy, and sincere in their belief that only through a power outside themselves could they remain abstinent. He had arrived in A.A. out of desperation, and determined that if it required belief in a God to get better, he would do it, because nothing else had worked for him, and this appeared to work for the others. He hated himself, but they accepted him just as he was, one of them. It was out of this acceptance that hope grew, for if these people who had reclaimed their lives accepted him, maybe he had some worth. The path was not specifically described, but he was told to get honest, to work the Steps, and to start to pray. He remained sober, and began to witness how he was being helped, but also how his experience was of benefit to others. As he persevered and worked the program amazing things began to happen which he could only explain as the result of a Higher Power working directly in his life. This supported his belief, and resulted in a determined effort to incorporate spiritual discipline into his daily life. He now describes this spiritual inquiry and practice as the single most important aspect of his existence.

Spiritual discipline is a vital aspect of any religious or spiritual tradition. It is also the hallmark of a solid Twelve Step program for the individual member. This practice, "working the Steps," is synonymous with daily attention to one's spiritual condition, an essential discipline. For most members the discipline involves both action and thought. It is a form of a cognitive behavioral approach that encourages examination of personal behavior through the filter of a Higher Power. One is asked to examine thoughts and behavior as they compare to that which they believe would be acceptable to this Higher Power. As mentioned, this involves prayer and meditation as well as using other group members as sounding boards for decision making. It places the individual's wishes in a secondary position to the spiritual path they have chosen, as to ignore this prioritization may result in relapse and the horror of addiction. By following these principles one not only remains abstinent, but begins to address the guilt and shame of addiction, establishes a renewed sense of self, and experiences the gifts of recovery. These gifts are documented in "the Promises," found in A.A.'s Big Book: "If we are painstaking about this phase of our development, we will be amazed before we are half way through. We are going to know a new freedom and a new happiness. We will not regret the past nor wish to shut the door on it. We will comprehend the word serenity and we will know peace. No matter how far down the scale we have gone, we will see how our experience can benefit others. That feeling of uselessness and self-pity will slip away. Our whole attitude and outlook upon life will change. Fear of people and economic insecurity will leave us. We will intuitively know how to handle situations which used to baffle us. We will suddenly realize that God is doing for us what we could not do for ourselves.''

REFERENCES

1. *Alcoholics Anonymous* (New York: Alcoholics Anonymous World Services, Inc., 1976) p. 83.
2. *Alcoholics Anonymous* (New York: Alcoholics Anonymous World Services, Inc., 1976) p. 25.
3. Ernest Kurtz, *Not-God: A History of Alcoholics Anonymous* (Center City, MN: Hazelden, 1979) pp. 3–4.
4. Ernest Kurtz, *Not-God: A History of Alcoholics Anonymous* (Center City, MN: Hazelden, 1979) p. 222.
5. *Alcoholics Anonymous* (New York: Alcoholics Anonymous World Services, Inc., 1976) p. 85.
6. *Alcoholics Anonymous* (New York: Alcoholics Anonymous World Services, Inc., 1976) p. 47.
7. *Alcoholics Anonymous* (New York: Alcoholics Anonymous World Services, Inc., 1976) p. 84.

3

Chapter Three

The Historical Perspective

In *Not-God*, Ernest Kurtz described four founding moments to the
A.A. movement: Dr. Carl Jung's involvement with Rowland H.;
Ebby T.'s November 1934 visit with Bill Wilson; Bill Wilson's
"spiritual experience" and his use of William James's *The
Varieties of Religious Experience*; and the interaction of Bill Wilson
and Dr. Bob Smith from May through June 10, 1935, which A.A.
considers its founding moment. Chapter Two describes the role of
Ebby T. and the initial involvement of Bill W. with Dr. Bob. This
chapter will document the other important moments and people
in a brief history of A.A. and Twelve Step programs.

Rowland H., a man of financial means, suffered from severe
alcoholism and had pursued numerous treatment attempts, all of
which had failed. He went to Zurich, Switzerland in 1931 to meet
with Dr. Carl Jung, the noted psychiatrist, believing that therapy
could bring him relief. They met for a year, and Rowland returned
to the US thinking that he was cured. He quickly relapsed, and
once again sought out Dr. Jung who informed Rowland that he
had a serious problem that no medical or psychiatric treatment
was known to cure. Essentially, Dr. Jung told him that he had a
hopeless condition. But Dr. Jung added that there was, perhaps,
one slim chance: a "spiritual awakening" or religious experience,
though the physician added that these were thought to be extremely rare events. Rowland H. was determined to find an answer, however, and he sought out the Oxford Group in England. When he

returned to New York, he continued his involvement with the American leader of the movement, Dr. Samuel Shoemaker, at the Calvary Episcopal Church.

The Oxford Group was started in 1908 by Frank Buchman, a Lutheran minister from Pennsylvania who had his own "spiritual experience" and was committed to bringing this to others, especially in academic settings, with an attempt to address worldly problems by personal spiritual change. It had a non-denominational, evangelical focus. The Oxford Group meetings were informal, often in members' homes, and emphasized fellowship. They did not require leaving one's own church, but assisted individuals in leading a Christian moral life. They worked toward a "changed life" by practicing specific principles. These included Five C's: confidence, confession, conviction, conversion, and continuance. They also practiced Five Procedures: give in to God; listen to God's directions; check guidance; restitution; and sharing (telling one's sins). The Oxford Group emphasized helping others to change, and in doing so recognizing personal benefits. They also refused to be paid for such work with others. The early A.A. experience was highly influenced by these principles, but much later Bill Wilson readily admitted that the A.A. founders gained knowledge of beneficial practices as well as recognition of some things to avoid. The Four Absolutes (absolute honesty, absolute purity, absolute unselfishness, absolute love) were considered too perfectionist for the recovering alcoholic who was so easily drawn into extremes of behavior. Kurtz summarized four "negative contributions" of the Oxford Group in the formation of A.A.: "Alcoholics Anonymous steadfastly and consistently rejected absolutes, avoided aggressive evangelism, embraced anonymity, and strove to avoid offending anyone who might need its program."[1]

While involved in the Oxford Group, Rowland H. remained abstinent. He practiced their principles and upon learning that an old friend was being threatened with a jail sentence for an alcohol-related offense, he paid him a visit. Ebby T. was dramatically influenced by Rowland's description of his ability to remain abstinent by involvement in the Oxford Group. When Ebby's sentence was stayed, he began to attend their meetings, and remained free of alcohol. He too followed their principles and sought out a friend and fellow drunk, Bill Wilson, to share what he had gained. Bill W. had been hospitalized at Charles B. Towns Hospital for the third time for the treatment of alcoholism on December 11, 1934. His extreme condition warranted discussion of commitment to a psychiatric facility. Ebby visited him during this round of detoxification and again described his own remarkable story. It was at this point that Bill W. had what he later described as a "hot flash," a sudden dramatic spiritual experience. He was in the midst of alcohol withdrawal and on medication to ease his condition, two factors that could have altered his consciousness. His experience was so unnatural that he was unsure whether he had had a hallucination or a profound awakening to something much greater than he had experienced up to this point in his life. In working with alcoholics and while starting the A.A. program with Dr. Bob Smith, Bill Wilson was hesitant to discuss this experience as he learned that it undermined his credibility, but much later he described it in detail at the "Alcoholics Anonymous Comes of Age" convention in 1955: "My depression deepened unbearably and finally it seemed to me as though I were at the bottom of a pit. I still gagged badly on the notion of a Power greater than myself, but finally, just for the moment, the last vestige of my proud obstinacy was crushed. All at once I found myself crying out, 'If there is a God let Him show Himself! I am ready to do anything, anything!' Suddenly the room lit up with a great white light. I was caught up into an ecstasy which there are no words to describe. It seemed to me, in the mind's eye, that I was on a mountain and that a wind not of air but of spirit was blowing. And then it burst upon me that I was a free man. Slowly the ecstasy subsided. I lay on the bed, but now for a time I was in another world, a new world of consciousness. All about me and through me there was a wonderful feeling of Presence, and I thought to myself, 'So this is the God of the preachers!' A great peace stole over me and I thought, 'No matter how wrong things seem to be, they are all right. Things are all right with God and His world.' "[2] Wilson sought out his psychiatrist, Dr. William Silkworth, to ask if he was going insane. Dr. Silkworth examined him, pronounced him perfectly sane, and described it as a "conversion experience." This supported Ebby T.'s Oxford Group experiences to which Bill had just begun to open himself and thus began to cement the spiritual foundation of his understanding of a new path to sobriety.

Dr. William Silkworth was medical director of Charles B. Towns Hospital, which specialized in the treatment of alcoholism and drug addiction. He was convinced that alcoholics had a physical vulnerability to alcohol. He described alcoholism in medical terms: "This is compulsion, this is pathological craving, this is disease" and "an obsession of the mind that condemns one to drink and an allergy of the body that condemns one to die."[3] He was convinced by his experience of treating over 50,000 alcoholics that this was a hopeless disease, but admitted that a "psychic change" could result in recovery. He also recognized the necessity of one alcoholic talking to another, and advised Bill to avoid preaching, but to describe the physical aspects of their disease. Dr. Silkworth believed this to be an inherent, chronic illness, and helped to set the initial understanding of the disease concept of alcoholism. This medical information was essential to the foundation of A.A., as Bill W. agreed that alcoholics could never drink safely.

Bill Wilson was immediately changed by his spiritual experience, and sought understanding of it. Ebby T. provided him a copy of William James's *The Varieties of Religious Experience*. It is the only book referenced in *Alcoholics Anonymous*. James's descriptions of conversion experiences and the ability to surrender after experiences of great pain contributed to Bill's beliefs. Bill W. later spoke of "deflation at depth" being a necessity for a spiritual experience. Ernest Kurtz points out that the influence of Silkworth and James resulted in two themes essential to the founding of the A.A. movement: "the hopelessness of the condition of the alcoholic, and the necessity of an experience of conversion."

After the hospitalization, Bill Wilson attended Oxford Group meetings, remained sober, and began his work with other alcoholics. He considered formal attempts to help alcoholics, but during his first six months of this effort he found no one else able to remain abstinent. It was during this period that Dr. Silkworth implored him to quit preaching and limit his discussions of his spiritual experience. He suggested emphasizing the medical facts and the hopelessness of the disease. In May 1935 Bill W. went to Akron and met Dr. Bob. Dr. Bob later described Bill W. as "the first living human with whom I had ever talked who knew what he was talking about in regard to alcoholism from actual experience." That summer Bill moved into Dr. Bob's home and together they pursued active alcoholics. The contrast of Bill's many failures in dealing with alcoholics and the success he shared with Dr. Bob resulted in the genesis of a plan that included "deflation at depth," sharing with another alcoholic to help one's self, and the use of the Oxford Group principles of spiritual growth.

Bill returned to New York in late summer 1935, and started another group of alcoholics within the Oxford Group. Thus their attempt to help alcoholics now had two distinct groups, one in New York and one in Akron. They remained subgroups of Oxford Groups but were not wholeheartedly accepted, especially in New York. Bill W. and Dr. Bob were in regular communication as they experimented with rules and regulations to help support the alcoholic's ability to remain abstinent. The tension between the alcoholic and nonalcoholic Oxford Group members grew, and in 1937, the alcoholics in the New York group split off to try to focus on alcoholism while maintaining a spiritual emphasis. That same year a group began in Cleveland that showed that Bill W. and Dr. Bob's methods could transfer to an independent location without one of the cofounders directly involved. In 1939, the Akron group left their Oxford Group as well. These early group meetings used Oxford Group teachings and practices, but had a singleness of purpose: sustained abstinence from alcohol.

The fledgling movement had to deal with many temptations, especially with Bill Wilson, a stockbroker, at the helm. Bill was offered a job as a lay counselor at Charles B. Towns Hospital, and there were thoughts of the A.A. founders starting their own hospitals for alcoholics, as well as treatment programs and other for-profit group activities. These ideas did not flourish as the membership realized the importance of their mission, and believed that the profit motive could undermine their program. The members disagreed with every new money making idea that Bill W. proposed. At one point they pursued financial backing from John D. Rockefeller, but he wisely refused. He did provide $5,000 to cover Bill W.'s mortgage and give a small monthly stipend to both Bill and Dr. Bob. This was extremely helpful, for they had no real income as they spent their time and resources helping alcoholics and devoting themselves to this new program. The meeting with John D. Rockefeller and other influential businessmen did result in other benefits, however, as they influenced the group of alcoholics to establish a board of directors. This resulted in the Alcoholic Foundation in 1938, a group composed of alcoholics and nonalcoholics. By 1954, the General Service Board had replaced the Alcoholic Foundation.

In 1938 Bill W. began to write a book to document their method of addressing people with serious alcohol problems. *Alcoholics Anonymous*, often referred to as the "Big Book," has two sections: a description of the A.A. program and stories of A.A. members. The title the founders chose for the book became the name of both the text and the organization. The book was written to bring their message to a much wider audience, but A.A. was nonetheless very slow to catch on. Writing *Alcoholics Anonymous* required that the founders organize and document their experiences; it also led to the establishment of the Twelve Steps. Bill W. attributed the Twelve Steps to influences from three sources: (1) the Oxford Group, (2) Dr. William Silkworth, (3) William James.[4] The Steps and much of the book were vigorously debated by the membership, which helped to shape them into their present form.

A.A. experienced slow but steady growth; by 1939 there were 100 people actively involved. After Akron, New York, and Cleveland, meetings sprang up in other Midwestern and East Coast cities. The members had expected a major response to the Big Book, but its impact was limited until they received some unsolicited publicity. A *Liberty* magazine article in 1939 resulted in 800 inquiries. There followed a series of articles in the Cleveland *Plain Dealer*. The most famous and influential article about the A.A. movement was by Jack Alexander in the *Saturday Evening Post* on March 1, 1941. This generated an enormous response that supported growth from 2,000 to 8,000 members during that year.

Dr. Harry M. Tiebout, a psychiatrist, became interested in A.A. after reading a pre-publication copy of *Alcoholics Anonymous*. He became an advocate of A.A. and advanced A.A.'s standing in the professional community. He arranged for Bill Wilson to speak on A.A. to the New York Medical Society and at a meeting of the American Psychiatric Association. This talk was published in the *American Journal of Psychiatry*. Dr. Tiebout supported the spiritual approach of A.A., and published articles on A.A. and alcoholism treatment.

With A.A.'s growth came conflict, and the cofounders spent much of their time addressing problems inherent to such a loosely run organization. Independent meetings popped up which were run by newly sober alcoholics. Bill W. recognized the potential for calamity and established a code of operation for the meetings. He developed the Twelve Traditions in an attempt to resolve problems and add structure to the self-governed meetings. He personally answered letters from A.A. members for years, responding to questions about A.A. and the meetings. A.A. started a newsletter in 1944, the *A.A. Grapevine*, to provide information to the membership. This publication served as a forum for the founders to address the membership and to define the evolving A.A. program over time. Bill wrote the book *Twelve Steps and Twelve Traditions* to further document A.A. principles.

Applying the A.A. program to people addicted to other drugs was considered by the early 1940s. Bill W. wrote about the dangers of drugs, calling them "goof balls" in an article in the *Grapevine* in 1945. In spite of this attention to other addictive substances Wilson maintained a strict stance that limited A.A.'s mission to alcoholics. Narcotics Anonymous (N.A.) was started between 1947 and 1953. Confusion in regard to the exact date exists due to several simultaneous efforts occurring around the US. There is documentation of a group called Addicts Anonymous beginning in February 1947 at the Federal Narcotics Hospital in Lexington, Kentucky. They based their meetings on A.A. principles, and Addicts Anonymous spread to other federal prisons, but it disappeared in the 1960s. The first official N.A. meeting occurred in 1949, arranged by Danny C. who had been involved in Addicts

Anonymous in Lexington. The initial meeting was at a Salvation Army cafeteria in New York. The New York group had dissolved by the early 1970s, but other groups had started in California in the 1950s. Jimmy K. is considered to be the founder of N.A. He and other founding members had close affiliations with A.A., and incorporated the Twelve Steps and Twelve Traditions into N.A. N.A. had more than 250,000 members by 1990.[5] The two programs are remarkably similar, using basically the same types of meetings and literature. N.A. uses the word addiction rather than alcohol in its first step. This signifies an inclusive stance in regard to abstinence from all drugs, including alcohol.

Bill Wilson was the driving force that shaped the A.A. program and every Twelve Step program to use these principles. He devoted his life to helping alcoholics, and after playing his tremendous role in A.A., consistently searched for new ways to help those who were unable to benefit from the A.A. program. He repeatedly avoided personal ambition to advance A.A. His cofounder, Dr. Bob Smith, played a less active role, yet he grounded the A.A. program with a stable, cautious approach that complemented the entrepreneurial energy of his partner. By working to save themselves they developed a program of spiritual principles that became the international hallmark in addressing alcoholism, and launched the other Twelve Step programs, helping millions of people with addictive behaviors.

REFERENCES

1. Ernest Kurtz, *Not-God: A History of Alcoholics Anonymous* (Center City, MN: Hazelden, 1979) p. 50.
2. Bill Wilson, *Alcoholics Anonymous Comes of Age* (New York: Alcoholics Anonymous World Services, Inc., 1957) p. 63.
3. *A.A. Grapevine* 7:12 99 (May 1951).
4. Bill Wilson, *The Language of the Heart: Bill W.'s Grapevine Writings* (New York: A.A. Grapevine, Inc., 1988).
5. Bob Stone, *My Years with Narcotics Anonymous: The History of N.A.* (Joplin, MO: Hulon Pendleton Publishing, 1997).

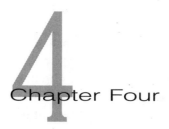

Chapter Four

Honesty

Honesty is considered to be an essential concept critical to the process of recovery from addiction. It can be thought of as a cornerstone to working a Twelve Step program. The importance of honesty to the individual in early recovery is often unrecognized by professionals, especially those unfamiliar with Twelve Step programs. We often only recognize the most blatant acts of dishonesty, as we tend to take most people at their word. This can be a significant mistake with people who are still active in their addiction, or even those in early recovery. Dishonesty and denial are considered the most consistent and persistent characteristics of people entering addiction treatment and Twelve Step programs. As health care providers we must recognize that we could be gaining inaccurate information, regularly, from this group. Collateral information and actual documented behavior must be used in the evaluation of the information provided by addicts. Clinicians must also be careful to address dishonesty as a symptom, and like any other, indicative of the disease. It is too convenient to dismiss people as lying drug addicts or alcoholics rather than to see them as having addictive disease with associated dishonesty. Most people with addictions have the ability to reestablish honesty, with self and with others, as they work a Twelve Step program, and health care workers can be of help in this process.

Honesty is considered a lost quality during active addiction, as people with these diseases have a tremendous capacity to lie to themselves. Some of this is in the form of denial, but there is also a tremendous degree of active manipulation. Maintenance of addictive behavior results in a self-centered sense of survival. The individual has established a new set of priorities in which maintaining the addiction is primary; for the addict, continuation of the addictive behavior is absolutely necessary. Thus, if lying is required to maintain the behavior, it may not be seen as much of a compromise. As this is repeated, one accommodates to the guilt and shame normally associated with dishonesty. This allows for repetition of the addictive behavior, and establishes denial. Some people lose the ability to witness the results of their behavior for they are lost in self-absorption. Most can only witness their destruction briefly, barely acknowledging the consequences of their behavior, which allows them to repeat it. Once the addictive pattern is established the individual uses whatever means necessary to avoid public disclosure. Dishonesty becomes the norm and begins to generalize, so that a lack of honesty begins to show up in other life spheres as well. It can become habitual, almost automatic, leaving the individual with an inability to converse naturally. Once this is established addicts lose the ability to honestly share themselves with others; every conversation is clouded by the dishonesty as well as associated shame and guilt. Addicts in this position may lie about their use of drugs and alcohol, but they may just as readily lie about their jobs, their relationships, and even inconsequential aspects of their lives.

Not surprisingly, friends and family members have great difficulty tolerating this degree of dishonesty; even the uninitiated recognize that a major problem exists. Addicts lose the trust that is associated with these relationships and, ultimately, the ability to trust themselves. Addicted individuals find that they cannot necessarily predict their own behavior, nor can they explain it to others. This results in ongoing attempts to justify and account for maladaptive behavior. In most families daily use of a psychoactive substance would not be tolerated. For the active addict this requires an excuse, a daily rationale, in order to avoid others while engaging in substance use. Most often they will not get caught, and the family will be unaware of the level of dishonesty and the extent of addictive behavior, but eventually people take note and are forced to confront the problem. Most families are caught unaware of the significance of an addiction because addicts have tremendous motivation to cover up their behavior. Once people realize the extent of the problem they often feel betrayed, and if they have witnessed repeated difficulties may find themselves with little ability to support the addict. Health care professionals can be faced with a similar situation, when individuals attempt to repeatedly procure drugs needed for addictive use. The physician will often refuse to prescribe without any attempt to promote treatment for the addiction. He or she may be angry with or disappointed in the addict, and express this, without recognizing the opportunity to intervene. It is often easier to react to the situation than to look beyond the symptom, dishonesty, and address the illness.

Denial is considered a subconscious defense mechanism. During active addiction denial allows maladaptive behavior to continue unchecked because addicted individuals lack the ability to examine themselves and cannot witness their behavior as problematic. Lay people often consider dishonesty a conscious act, however. Twelve Step programs do not distinguish between the two, nor do they define dishonesty in their literature. They simply say the addict needs to "get honest"; Twelve Step programs are self-described as "honesty programs." The assumption is that most addicts still maintain an internal sense of right and wrong, of honesty and dishonesty. Honesty may not be defined, but it is readily recognized. New members are faced with living examples of people who have willingly examined their behavior, admitted extreme problems, and even discuss them publicly. The new member learns that it is unacceptable to use the subconscious (denial) as an excuse, or a reason for his or her troubles. He or she also learns that other members have had their own experiences with dishonesty and are not easily fooled. The emphasis on honesty can be quite shocking for addicts new to recovery, yet it sets the stage for their initial attempts to open up and truthfully share their stories, to describe what brought them to the meetings. Denial and dishonesty are quickly confronted in addiction treatment programs. This is not necessarily the case in Twelve Step programs where it is believed that while honesty is required, it takes time. Dishonesty is accepted in the newcomer, but only in the knowledge that working the program will, over time, effectively address the denial and the dishonesty. "The antidote for the deep symptom of denial was identification marked by open and undemanding narration infused with profound honesty about personal witness."[1]

Active participation in a Twelve Step group is considered the beginning of a process of self-acceptance. This act results in the admission of a problem, which is necessary for the addict to enter into recovery, and establishes for the individual the first glimpse of the truth of his or her condition. It is believed that the ability to get honest with oneself is required to adequately work the Steps, which require an in-depth examination of thoughts and behavior. Honesty is not a frank prerequisite to the Steps, but it is considered necessary to working the Steps as they are intended to be worked; that is, in a manner that will result in the "spiritual awakening" described in Step Twelve and in attaining the "promises" as elucidated in the Big Book. The treatment of addictions can be considered, at its most basic level, an attempt to encourage this type of honest self-appraisal that results in recognition of the consequences that have befallen the individual as a result of this disease.

Honesty is explicitly emphasized in Twelve Step meetings; integrity is modeled and expected. The act of attending meetings reveals at least some recognition of the need for help. Attending meetings and listening to how those with long-term sobriety grapple with honest self-appraisal, newly recovering addicts begin to emerge from the blinding effects of denial to clearly witness their inner lives and their behavior. This type of self-examination precedes the ability to face and open up to others, which marks the initial stages of recovery. The first paragraph of the fifth chapter of *Alcoholics Anonymous*, which precedes the documentation of the Twelve Steps, reveals a strict, explicit emphasis on honesty as a requirement to recovery. "Rarely have we seen a person fail who has thoroughly followed our path. Those who do not recover are people who cannot or will not completely give themselves to this simple program, usually men and women who are constitutionally incapable of being honest with themselves. There are such unfortunates. They are not at fault; they seem to have been born that way. They are naturally incapable of grasping and developing a manner of living which demands rigorous honesty. Their chances are less than average. There are those, too, who suffer from grave emotional and mental disorders, but many of them do recover if they have the capacity to be honest."[2]

In the context of a Twelve Step meeting honesty is emphasized and modeled in the remarkable stories of the experience of addiction that are told by the members. These stories are an attempt to express the reality of the addictive lifestyle, with all its pain and consequences, for the individual and the group. Much of what is described would be unacceptable in other forums, and most people are reticent to even begin to share such damaging tales, but when they witness the stories of others, and the acceptance of the behaviors as "normal" to the addictive experience, it allows them to begin to release publicly that which they do not even want to examine in private. This level of acceptance of the behaviors, the problems, and the unspoken acts, is a powerful, reinforcing agent of change. "The therapeutic power of this process of identification arose from the witness it gave, a witness to the healing potency of the shared honesty of mutual vulnerability openly acknowledged. The healing response to this invitation, this witness, lay in the act of surrender—the necessary foundation for 'getting the program' of Alcoholics Anonymous."[1]

The surrender Kurtz discusses is inherent to the active participation in a Twelve Step program. This level of surrender is an act of acceptance that one has a severe illness, and that there is a solution to be found in this "simple program," a solution based in spiritual principles. This acknowledgment begins the process of breaking through the denial that maintains the addiction itself. To successfully address the addictive thought patterns requires the "rigorous honesty" referred to in the A.A. text. It also requires a group experience in which acceptance by others results in acceptance of self. Only consistent efforts to witness the truth about one's behavior and the attributes of this illness will prevent the insidious return of self-deception, and with it the denial and dishonesty that would allow the addiction to become active again. Inherent in the telling of these stories of the addictive experience is the expectation that this will keep people clean and sober. It is an act of release, an act of freedom, from the secret horrors of addiction. Honesty is considered essential to the process of recovery.

"To thine own self be true" is a phrase common to Twelve Step meetings. It is used to remind members to continue efforts to eliminate self-deception. Even addicts in recovery struggle with honesty; the resolution of long-standing dishonesty is not quick or easy. In fact, this can be an ongoing problem that undermines the individual's ability to adequately work the Steps, limiting the personal growth inherent to this process. There is, of course, a simplicity in the truth; maintaining one's perspective in reality requires little or no exaggeration or manipulation. Yet this can be very difficult for active or newly recovering addicts to grasp. People in early recovery have a very poor understanding of honest thought and interaction, and they often require the assistance of others in the pursuit of the truth for themselves. For this reason it is recommended that members regularly share with others, and use a sponsor in examining these issues of personal truth. Humans can convince themselves of almost anything, but in discussion with peers, in gaining the perspective of formulating ideas for others as well as accepting someone else's views and feedback, the individual can begin to grow in understanding of honesty. Behavioral methods are incorporated in this process as well. Members practice making their word their bond and simply doing what they say they will. In Twelve Step programs people discuss ongoing efforts to avoid secrets as they work on honesty, and attempt to share themselves with others in a manner that protects against self-deception. One key A.A. aphorism is, "You're only as sick as your secrets." The process of eliminating denial and making a priority of honesty are required to work the Twelve Steps and allow for a new way of life to begin.

This above all: to thine own self be true,
And it must follow, as the night the day,
Thou canst not then be false to any man.
                    William Shakespeare, *Hamlet*

REFERENCES

1. Ernest Kurtz, *Not-God: A History of Alcoholics Anonymous* (Center City, MN: Hazelden, 1979) p. 61.
2. *Alcoholics Anonymous* (New York: Alcoholics Anonymous World Services, Inc., 1976) p. 58.

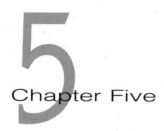

Chapter Five

Step One

"We admitted we were powerless over alcohol—that our lives
had become unmanageable."

Step One is considered a statement of the problem. It is the admission that a problem exists, and this admission is essential to the initiation of the recovery process. A deep level of acceptance that requires honest self-appraisal and breaking through denial precedes this type of admission. This is the only step to mention drugs, alcohol or the addictive behavior. It should be noted that Step One does not state, "Quit doing this, then do this." It is not a prerequisite to stop the addictive pattern before working the rest of the Steps. The expectation is that one will hit bottom, seek an answer to the problem in this program, and quit the addictive behavior as a result of this process. The two features of this Step that must be examined by the individual are powerlessness and unmanageability. These are not synonymous: powerlessness is considered the "out of control" behavior of the individual, the addiction itself, while unmanageability is described in terms of the consequences of the behavior to the individual and to others.

This is an extremely difficult step for people to take, but it is fundamental to the entire process as it sets the stage for life change that cannot occur without recognition of the dire *need* to change. On the surface it would appear to be an obvious statement, a simple description of the problem at hand. Addictions exercise incredible power over people, becoming their primary drive. This results in extreme resistance to intervention and limits the ability of the person to admit to the need for help. In addressing Step

One, the A.A. text *Twelve Steps and Twelve Traditions* states: "Who cares to admit complete defeat?" This idea is reiterated in *Narcotics Anonymous*: "Help for addicts begins only when we are able to admit complete defeat." To examine oneself in this manner usually requires "hitting bottom." This refers to reaching a point, as the result of negative consequences sufficiently painful, where a person will begin to admit the need for change and perhaps even the need for help. This suggests a breakdown in denial of the problem that provides enough of a glimpse of reality to result in honest evaluation of the depth of the problem.

Most people do not want to admit defeat, or to change, when they begin to examine themselves and their behavior as it relates to the addiction. Unless they truly hit a bottom, they will not see this as an insurmountable problem; in fact, they may have many ideas about minor changes that they think will be adequate to fix the problem. A true addiction will not respond to such attempts, though addicts will readily fool themselves into believing it will. Professionals have to be careful not to fall into this trap, as it is difficult to grasp the true depth and power of an addiction, and the afflicted will have sound rationale for their alternative attempts at change. Often they will look for the "reason" for the addiction, which is certainly tempting for any therapist. The alcoholic is always looking for the way out, the way they ended up like this, the external factor that makes them so miserable. It is easy to blame it on peripheral problems as so many will exist related to the addictive behavior. Addicts would much rather find fault in their job, their marriage or their upbringing than admit that they may be the problem. They will try to find the "reason," rather than look at themselves and their substance use. Clinicians will repeatedly hear active addicts say, "If I could just [do this], I could stay clean and sober." "This" is always an external problem or a minor behavioral change that could possibly enhance their lives in some manner, and is related to the underlying problem, but will not, even if addressed, adequately deal with the addiction. Step One focuses the individual on the problem, and emphasizes that the responsibility for the situation is with the addict alone. John M. may have put it best when he said simply, "John's problem is

John." As long as one is searching for an external answer or an underlying reason, one does not have to examine the real problem. This allows for ongoing alcohol or drug use.

Internally the addict must recognize the inability to drink and drug like most people, admit the problem, and eliminate rationalizations for ongoing use, which manifest in a tendency to look for exceptions that suggest the possibility of controlled use. The power of the addiction to sway rational thought processes, combined with significant denial, results in some very suspect reasoning that supports ongoing use. Addicts tend to develop their own definitions of addiction. In this manner they prevent admission of the problem by never meeting their often-shifting criteria for what constitutes addiction. Chemical dependency professionals deal with people who believe they could only be addicted if they went to jail, if their use affected their work, if they used as much as their fathers had, if they were living on the streets, and so on. Some people use a different approach. They say they are alcoholic but never truly admit to powerlessness or unmanageability. They seem to readily identify the problem, but in truth they hang onto rationalizations that convince themselves that they still have control. These and other means of avoiding the truth about the addictive behavior allow for ongoing use, and Twelve Step programs state that a bottom must be reached to open the individual's mind to the reality of the situation. "Many less desperate alcoholics tried A.A., but did not succeed because they could not make the admission of hopelessness."[1]

Regarding Step One, the N.A. text states: "Powerlessness means doing drugs against your will." This is a strong but accurate statement. To be powerless also means to continue the addiction in spite of adverse consequences. Obvious problems exist that are specifically related to a pattern of drug and alcohol use, but the addict can do nothing to alter the course of the illness. This can be a very lonely, hopeless condition. Addicts find themselves caught in a position in which they are able to recognize the need to stop, but also know that they cannot do it. They need to surrender, to "admit defeat," in order to begin the process of recovery, yet it goes against their nature to do so. Therapists often minimize powerlessness, perceiving the problem as poor effort or a lack of effort in controlling a certain behavior. They do not understand the true power of the addiction, which effects a change in priority of drive states in which the addiction takes precedence over the addict's very survival. This results in the absolute inability of the individual to alter the addictive behavior patterns. It usually does not appear this dire, however, and it may be easy for the clinician to convince him or herself that it is not. Just as addicts erroneously perceive control, clinicians may mistakenly attribute control to them. But any disease must be examined on a continuum. Diabetes does not seem so bad when well managed and no physiologic consequences have begun, but it is nightmarish when one has lost a foot to amputation, is blind, and is losing kidney function. At end stage disease, addiction, like any life-threatening illness, is easy to recognize, but what we often do not recognize is that the early interventions have to be based in the recognition of powerlessness. In the midst of addiction people look and act insane; they hurt themselves and loved ones in order to continue the addictive behavior. They do not engage in these acts due to a lack of intelligence or a lack of compassion. It is not a conscious decision to self-destruct. They are powerless to do anything else. The anesthesiologist who dumps out the sharps box, full of bio-hazardous waste, and sifts through it with bare hands trying to find a few drops of fentanyl, does not lack for intellect, he lacks control. The nurse who fixes her heroin with toilet water does not lack an understanding of the risk, she lacks control. The alcoholic who leaves her two-year-old alone while she goes out for "just one" but does not come back for three days, does not lack love and compassion for the child, she lacks control. They are powerless to do anything else; they are controlled by their addiction. "The foundation of our program is the admission that we, of ourselves, do not have power over addiction."[2]

Twelve Step members regard unmanageability as the negative consequences of their addictive behavior. They examine these consequences in Step One to continue the task of breaking through denial and viewing the reality of the addiction. Out of control behavior results in damage to self and others. The dual aspect of Step One reveals to the individual that he or she has no control over the addiction, and this has resulted in considerable damage. It is easy to examine the consequences that are directly related to intoxication. People often begin by admitting to the facts: falls, broken bones, fights, car accidents, driving under the influence, divorce, lost friendships, cellulitis, HIV, hepatitis, and so on. Secondary consequences are related more to deterioration of functioning than directly to intoxication. The member examines problems that effect family, academic achievement, job performance, finances, and social activities. Less obvious are abstract consequences, those that involve the addict's emotional stability, personal growth, expectations, and goals. As these consequences expand, a loss of identity occurs, leaving the individual with a radically diminished self-concept. Negative consequences undermine the individual's dignity, while denial and dishonesty displace integrity. Guilt and shame expand while self-confidence wanes. The individual is deteriorating in dramatic fashion, and at some level it is acknowledged, even as they are trying to deny it and avoid discovery by others. This is the true pain of addiction and requires either continued anesthesia, or frank admission to elicit the possibility of change.

Many of the problems examined as unmanageability are not directly related to the intoxicating effects of the addictive substance, but they are directly related to the disease. Once the addict is abstinent, many of these problems remain. Some A.A. members refer to this as the "ism" of alcoholism, suggesting that there is much more than abstinence that needs to be examined. Minor problems that precede addictive behavior are exaggerated during the years of active addiction. These problems do not get addressed, and thus they worsen and can become considerable deficits. People in Twelve Step programs may refer to an unmanageability that precedes active addiction for this reason. This can be understood in relation to the limited psychological development that occurs during addiction. If one sees intoxication as a numbing, powerful, coping mechanism, it is easy to recognize how regular use of a substance can eliminate the necessity of other coping skills. By default, the numbing secondary to intoxication becomes the major, if not only, coping strategy that is used by the individual. This eliminates formal development of other coping mechanisms that leaves the addict bare of such skills once they quit using drugs or alcohol. In addition, many addicts have poor pain tolerance due to the level of numbing that has been occurring, and they are thus quite sensitive to any psychic pain. Once clean and sober, addicts lose the only defense they had at their disposal, which can result in what appears to be a deterioration of emotional functioning. Initial sobriety can be extremely difficult as a result. The newly sober may have difficulty handling stressors that were quite readily handled in the past, even during the addiction.

Some newcomers and some therapists refute the Twelve Step understanding of unmanageability, especially as it relates to behavior preceding the addiction. They mistakenly argue that these programs blame all problems on the addiction. Honest examination of one's behavior in a manner indicative of the level of admission necessary to Step One will reveal consequences that are specific to addictive behavior as well as independent problems that are exaggerated by the disease. Negative behavioral patterns based in childhood experience may worsen during active addiction, but are not the result of the addiction. The Twelve Step view of unmanageability does not suggest that the addiction causes all of these problems, but it does recommend that the individual examine the numerous ways in which the addiction has negatively influenced their lives. The recognition of this relatedness, and acceptance of the depth of the addiction, is necessary to the process of admission.

Twelve Step members tell their "story" in meetings devoted to discussion of Step One using the simple format, "what it was like, what happened, and what it is like now."[3] Once the admission of powerlessness and unmanageability has occurred, people are readily able to describe the insanity of their use and the related patterns of behavior and do so in a graphic manner. These descriptions are often tragic, but they can also be comic, as members relate the ridiculous ways in which they acted while unaware of the depth of their problem. This is amusing to the indoctrinated who understand the tragedies to be in the past, almost a different life altogether, as the result of the personal gains they have made in recovery. In this, the newcomer hears an essential message: "I was out of control, but I didn't know it. Look at these familiar examples of the crazy, harmful things I did before I got here." The latter part of the message, which is often unspoken, is also pertinent, "and look at me now." These stories are the route to identification necessary to breaking through denial and acceptance of self as addict/alcoholic. Admission of the problem and identification with other members brings about hope, the possibility for change.

Treatment centers use Step One for the same purpose: to help people honestly admit that a problem exists with a level of understanding that can lead to recognition of the necessity for change. It is not about describing the sad story of one's life, the "bad breaks and misunderstandings" that resulted in entering treatment. Most people do not want to change, even when faced with major consequences. They cannot admit to powerlessness, and do not relate to unmanageability. They attempt to continue to grasp at the mirage of control. A helpful strategy described by one chemical dependency counselor is to have the individual list ten specific examples of attempts to control use that resulted in a failure to do so. This can elicit the reality of powerlessness, rather than the justification of intention. This counselor states that clients often struggle to come up with ten examples, so he suggests they ask their spouse or other family members to help them. These others can almost always readily describe numerous examples. Then the addict is asked to examine the impact of these episodes on different life spheres (vocational, emotional, physical, family, financial), specifically linking the powerlessness to consequences, in order to address unmanageability. People will often admit to significant consequences, without truly admitting to powerlessness, which leaves the door open to ongoing addictive behavior, a pitfall which the counselor—and the individual—must recognize. Properly executed, this attempt at breaking through denial to produce the admission associated with Step One is often successful, and is the foundation of treatment programs that use the Twelve Steps.

Step One is completed by identifying and admitting to the problem, an admission that results from hopelessness, not strength. People do not get to this point without significant difficulties, which must be faced with courage. The individual discovers the extent of the problem by examining his or her powerlessness and unmanageability and breaking through denial to view the reality of addiction. In this undertaking he or she begins to recognize their inability to use drugs and alcohol like other people and addresses the rationalizations that have prevented recognition of his or her plight. All members of Twelve Step groups understand the necessity of a thorough Step One. Without it, one is consistently battling thoughts that justify ongoing involvement in the addictive behavior, which often leads to relapse. Completion of Step One instills hope, and the possibility of change, which is directly related to the ability to identify with other members working a program. Twelve Step program members go on to speak of powerlessness and unmanageability in recovery, after abstinence is established, to reflect the necessity of ongoing attention to underlying problems. Abstinence is only the beginning of recovery; it is the necessary foundation for proper involvement in a spiritual program that can result in tremendous life change. This reveals the essence of the other Eleven Steps, as they are considered a blueprint for change. Only out of recognition, and hitting bottom, does admission of the problem occur, allowing one to move on to the healing process of recovery.

REFERENCES

1. *The Twelve Steps and Twelve Traditions* (New York: Alcoholics Anonymous World Services, Inc., 1988) p. 23.
2. *Narcotics Anonymous, 5th Ed.* (Van Nuys, CA: N.A. World Services, Inc., 1988) p. 21.
3. *Alcoholics Anonymous, 3rd Ed.* (New York: A.A. World Services, Inc., 1976) p. 58.

Chapter Six

Step Two

"Came to believe that a Power greater than ourselves could restore us to sanity."

Step Two summarizes the thoughts of the cofounders and early members of A.A. who found that the only solution to the problem defined in Step One is of a spiritual nature. Step One is a statement of the problem, whereas Step Two is a description of the solution, an indoctrination into the core spiritual beliefs of the Twelve Steps. There is no sudden solution or change associated with Step Two; it is only the beginning of a spiritual program, and can take months to fully realize. Addicts are faced with the hopelessness of their condition as defined by Step One yet continue to live a powerless and unmanageable existence. They are humbled by Step One, desperate for an answer, and ready for help. An old A.A. saying describes this progression into a spiritual examination of self: first we came, then we came to, then we came to believe. To paraphrase Kurtz, the A.A. member gains strength from the recognition of weakness, must admit that they are not-God, and look to a power outside themselves. "Remember that we deal with alcohol—cunning, baffling, powerful! Without help it is too much for us. But there is One who has all power—that One is God. May you find Him now!"[1]

Bill Wilson did not readily adopt a spiritual stance prior to his attempts to work with alcoholics. He was actually resistant to consideration of such an approach, until he witnessed the changes in his friend Ebby T., desperately sought a similar path, and experienced a sudden, dramatic spiritual experience (see Chapter 2).

His experience enabled him to recognize the predicament most people face when examining these Steps, but it also provided the necessary tools to develop a program that was inclusive in its approach, allowing people of remarkably different religious and spiritual backgrounds to come together and examine themselves using this simple program. He started the chapter devoted to Step Two in *Twelve Steps and Twelve Traditions* with a discussion of the difficulties people face after Step One, when they realize that A.A.'s solution is spiritual. "The moment they read Step Two, most A.A. newcomers are confronted with a dilemma, sometimes a serious one. How often have we heard them cry out, 'Look what you people have done to us! You have convinced us that we are alcoholics and that our lives are unmanageable. Having reduced us to a state of absolute helplessness, you now declare that none but a Higher Power can remove our obsession. Some of us would not believe in God, others can not, and still others who do believe that God exists have no faith whatever He will perform this miracle.'"

This truly is a dilemma for many newcomers, and for the therapists that work with them. How does one examine the elimination of addiction by looking to a Power greater than oneself? There is no definition or prescribed method for accomplishing this task; the Steps themselves are suggested, not required. This is a verbal tradition, shared in the form of personal stories specific to each Step. Veteran members of Twelve Step programs are often adept at addressing the Higher Power dilemma, because it is a frequent problem for newcomers; old-timers thus are willing and able to share their own struggles with this Step. Some people do not believe in anything, and refuse to give this Step much consideration; often they will, in fact, oppose such a perspective. Many have lost the beliefs they once had. The *Alcoholics Anonymous* text addresses such groups formally with a chapter entitled "We Agnostics," various excerpts for atheists, and ample stories of the difficulties people have with this Step. Many people have biases about religion, some religions exclude members of other religions, and some people cannot involve themselves in Twelve Step programs because of their religious beliefs. Twelve Step members have had to grapple with this Step and come to grips with its primary intent: the realization that individuals cannot heal themselves and need to rely on a Higher Power. The founders of A.A. worked to minimize the dilemma by placing the emphasis on spirituality, not religion, while maintaining the focus on a specific task, sobriety. "If you have decided you want what we have and are willing to go to any length to get it—then you are ready to take certain steps."[2]

Some people find it difficult to consider the restoration of sanity because they do not accept Step One, or they do not understand the intended concept. Twelve Step programs do not use definitions, but members normally speak of the insanity related to the addictive behavior, insanity exposed as the powerless and unmanageability of Step One. Sanity is described as "soundness of mind" in *Twelve Steps and Twelve Traditions*. The Narcotics Anonymous (N.A.) text states, "Insanity is repeating the same mistakes and expecting different results." If one does not recognize the insanity related to powerlessness and unmanageability, the concept of restoration is useless, and the individual may not be ready for involvement in a Twelve Step program. The ongoing use of a drug in spite of adverse consequences must be accepted as a form of insanity. This does not even begin to address the lies, manipulations, rationalizations, distortion of self-image, and deterioration of functioning associated with addiction. Some people focus on their unique situation to avoid examination of this Step: "I'm too far gone for help" or "I really don't have a problem like that." Some people do not want to admit they need help at all, making the admission of insanity impossible. The admission of Step One is a definite requirement that precedes the Second Step.

"True humility and an open mind can lead us to faith, and every A.A. meeting is an assurance that God will restore us to sanity if we rightly relate ourselves to Him."[3] Members of Twelve Step programs accept this description to be true, and they even have a saying specific to it: "act as if." As newcomers enter this program with the expectation of gaining help in mastering an addiction, little do they know that they will be asked to accept defeat and then gain strength from a Higher Power. If they can examine these concepts and keep an open mind, they will begin a life-long journey of recovery based in spiritual principles. The members are not asked to *define* a Power greater than themselves, they are asked to *believe*. The Step does not stop at mere belief though; the expectation is that this power will play a particular role in the life of the believer, a restoration of sanity. "Most of us lacked a working relationship with a Higher Power. We begin to develop this relationship by simply admitting to the possibility of a Power greater than ourselves."[4] This "working relationship" is a core principle of the Twelve Steps, a belief that a Higher Power will not only address the addiction, but play an active part in the achievement of healing and wholeness.

People gain hope in witnessing the remarkable changes this program has provided to the experienced members. The recognition of faith in others who speak of these Steps as the manner in which they have altered their life course can instill faith in the newcomer. Most people come to believe by witnessing positive changes in others who attribute these changes to a power greater than themselves. The demonstrations occur in the meetings, through discussions with other members, through the loving care of a sponsor, and by witnessing people using these principles to address any number of life's essential problems with an ease that reveals the belief associated with Step Two. "In A.A. we saw the fruits of this belief: men and women spared from alcohol's final catastrophe. We saw them meet and transcend their other pains and trials. We saw them calmly accept impossible situations, seeking neither to run nor to recriminate. This was not only faith; it was faith that worked under all conditions. We soon concluded that whatever price in humility we must pay, we would pay."[5] When a manipulative, dishonest newcomer hears the same stories of self-centeredness, deception, and disregard for others from the member with several years of sobriety who greeted him or her with open arms and seems to sincerely care about others, it can have a dramatic effect. The sharing of these stories provides the witness needed to establish hope for the possibility of change.

The newcomer begins to realize that change can actually occur and that there is help in this process—assistance from fellow Twelve Step members and from a Higher Power. Addiction is a lonely illness; people become very isolated and mistrustful. It is difficult for them to believe that others will actually help them, but the acceptance and support they experience from other members encourages a hopeful new stance. They realize they do not have to engage in this struggle alone, they are not hopeless, and their lives have meaning. Hope blossoms in the recognition of the possibility of change noted in the stories of other members, and it is supported by the the acceptance of others with their shared vision that anyone is deserving of what they have so freely received in these programs. The experienced members see themselves in the newcomer and are reminded of the horror of the disease. At the same time they continually witness the miracles of change, which begin when people "come to believe." These people provide the newcomer with a palpable degree of hope based on their own experiences with these Steps.

One member described his own struggle with Step Two. He had been brought up in a religion that no longer held any meaning for him. He viewed himself with great shame, as worthless, if not sub-human. Upon entering A.A. he was accepted by the other members, in spite of his own self-concept. They listened to him and seemed to care about him. Their stories matched his own in uncanny ways, and he began to believe that if they could stay sober perhaps he could too. He was attracted to discussions of the spirituality of the program, but had no idea what it meant. People talked of a Higher Power, as if they could actually count on it for help in staying sober and in dealing with everyday life. This did not match his understanding, and so while he listened to their experience, he found no evidence of such a Power. He appreciated that it did not have to be any particular God, especially not the God of his upbringing. He was able to begin to be honest with a select few, especially his sponsor. He admitted his fears, in particular that he may not make it. He read the literature, attended meetings, and followed his sponsor's advice. Yet, he could not grasp Step Two. In a way he overlooked it, deciding that he had a belief that something existed, but not recognizing the possibility that this Power would work in his daily life. Sobriety was a struggle; he regularly thought of using drugs and alcohol, and continued to have marked problems with responsibility and honesty. His irresponsibility resulted in a significant financial problem. He had promised to take two of his younger brothers on a canoe trip, but had run out of money again. His sponsor was a fairly wealthy guy, so he approached him with thoughts of describing how important this was, a manipulation that he hoped would result in an offer for a loan. He told his sponsor the tale, and was surprised when the sponsor asked, "Have you prayed about it?" This was unexpected, and he thought to himself that prayer could be of no help whatsoever. His sponsor repeated the question, and then suggested that it could be helpful. Although angry that he did not get what he wanted, he thought about his sponsor's recommendation. He mumbled some annoyed thoughts about how this seemed ridiculous, then said a simple prayer, with no belief that it would be worthwhile. He had no other options, so he repeated a prayer the next day, and the next. He respected his sponsor and had found that following his advice had been fruitful in the past, so he kept up this vigil. The irritating process had become easier, and he began to speak as if something was listening. The next week, just a couple days before the trip was to begin, he went to the mail and found his federal income tax return check. He was astonished, considered it a miracle, and still describes it as the foundation of belief that a Higher Power actually cared for him in the events of his daily life. This circumstance, this synchronicity, established the belief associated with Step Two and marked the beginning of a life devoted to spiritual principles.

Step Two is not just for newcomers. It is a Step that requires revisiting on a regular basis. Most spiritual disciplines recognize that belief can wane, requiring renewed commitment. The same is true for this program. It is very easy to forget the pain that brings people to a Twelve Step program, allowing one to begin to lose sight of the necessity of these Steps. This can certainly happen with the established member of a Twelve Step program. Insanity can return in many forms, it is not limited to active alcohol and drug use. People can become unmanageable in recovery, and may need to reexamine the role of the Second Step in their lives. The establishment of belief in a Higher Power does not suggest belief is everlasting. The most likely way in which one can forget the essence of this Step is in a diminishing belief that this Power will work in one's daily life. This can occur as one becomes healthier, more "normal," and less concerned with the crisis of the addictive process. For the newcomer, restoration of sanity may be much easier to consider as it relates to the consequences of drug and alcohol use than it is for the forty-five-year-old businesswoman who finds she is overworking, stressed out, and has developed a gastric ulcer. Both may need to examine this Step and begin a process of life change based on spiritual principles.

Professionals need to provide the client engaged in Step Two the room to struggle with it and develop his or her own concept of a Power greater than themselves. This difficult process must be honored as a sacred undertaking. Just as Twelve Step programs provide stories and experience related to this Step, the professional can provide examples of struggle with belief, using differing spiritual and religious perspectives. It is important to avoid expression of religious bias, and maintain the open, inclusive stance of Twelve Step spirituality. It can also be beneficial to engage the client in an examination of his or her past beliefs: what was the nature of their religious background, have they examined spiritual principles, have there been negative experiences, and do they consider this a legitimate effort. The individual is attempting to develop the foundation of a spiritual program but may not recognize this process as such an effort. The professional can make this an emphasis, present connections to other Steps, and provide examples of spiritual disciplines. The professional is also in an excellent position to provide legitimacy to the entire effort and to present an appropriate perspective on the idea of "insanity" referred to in Step Two. An understanding of the spiritual concepts of Twelve Step programs can provide the professional with a legitimate role in helping clients examine Step Two.

REFERENCES

1. *Alcoholics Anonymous, 3rd Ed.* (New York: A.A. World Services, Inc., 1976) pp. 58–59
2. *Alcoholics Anonymous, 3rd Ed.* (New York: A.A. World Services, Inc., 1976) p. 58.
3. *The Twelve Steps and Twelve Traditions* (New York: Alcoholics Anonymous World Services, Inc., 1988) p. 34.
4. *Narcotics Anonymous, 5th Ed.* (Van Nuys, CA: N.A. World Services, Inc., 1988) p. 23.
5. *The Twelve Steps and Twelve Traditions* (New York: Alcoholics Anonymous World Services, Inc., 1988) p. 32.

7

Chapter Seven

Step Three

"Made a decision to turn our will and our lives over to the care of God as we understood Him."

Step Three expands the notion of a Higher Power that works directly in the individual's life. It reveals the route by which the individual can alter thinking and, ultimately, behavior. It is described as the first of the action Steps, as this concept takes the person beyond belief and into direct action to initiate a remarkable change in perspective and conduct. "This is the way to a faith that works."[1] This Step is a statement of commitment to a spiritual path at a level not well understood by the initiate. It is not just a deepening of understanding it is a proclamation of a new way of life. Repeatedly making this "decision" results in surrender, recognition of limits, and an acceptance of the role that a Higher Power can take in daily life. It is an attempt to reach out for help with the expectation that a Higher Power can direct one's will and life in a manner that the individual is incapable of doing. It is a mystical Step, not readily obvious in its intent, which can confound the Twelve Step member. It requires further examination of a Higher Power—"God as we understood Him"—and begins the development of the practice of "turning it over." Working this Step places one on a spiritual path that seems to go against the grain of self-sufficiency, but actually provides a profound level of freedom and independence. This Step is the essence of a spiritual program, providing the Twelve Step member with the basics of spiritual discipline. "In fact, the effectiveness of the whole A.A. program will rest upon how well and earnestly we have tried to come to 'a decision to turn our will and our lives over to the care of God *as we understood Him.*'"[2]

The disaster of addiction recognized in Step One and the establishment of belief in Step Two seldom result in any change in the remarkably self-absorbed stance of the practicing alcoholic or addict. "Selfishness—self centeredness! That, we think, is the root of our troubles."[3] Step Three places the focus outside one's self, suggesting that recovery cannot be initiated if the individual's perspective remains the same, attempting to control themselves and their environs by their own willpower. "The first requirement is that we be convinced that any life run on self-will can hardly be a success."[4] Twelve Step programs acknowledge that the self-absorption that allows for addictive behavior to continue expands throughout the period of active use and can prevent the individual from making any useful life changes. If someone remains convinced that they have the answers, they have no ability to begin a spiritual path, and to see themselves as not-God. A sincere attempt to begin to work Step Three starts with the recognition that one's best thinking resulted in the calamity of active addiction, and that no lasting solution can be found on one's own. This Step presupposes the first two Steps. It requires a marked degree of humility, an understanding of human limitations, and, ultimately, a willingness to seek out a Higher Power. "So our troubles we think are basically of our own making. They arise out of ourselves, and the alcoholic is an extreme example of self will run riot, though he usually doesn't think so. Above everything, we alcoholics must get rid of our selfishness. We must, or it kills us! God makes that possible. And there often seems no way of entirely getting rid of self without His aid. Many of us had moral and philosophical convictions galore, but we could not live up to them even though we would have liked to. Neither could we reduce our self-centeredness much by wishing or trying on our own power. We had to have God's help ... First of all we had to quit playing God. It didn't work."[3]

Step Three expands upon the recognition of need for help noted in the Second Step, revealing a path that involves "turning over one's will and life." This is a spiritual act of letting go; it is mystical by nature, not defined but expected. As in so many aspects of these programs, the task is left up to the individual to discover just what it is that is expected for him or herself, with the help of their more experienced peers. Faith that a Higher Power will care for individual needs on a day-to-day basis is at the root of this Step. One cannot "turn it over" without such faith. The recovering person, depleted of coping skills, finds relief in this form of surrender. Excessive fear haunts the newcomer, worry about the past is overwhelming, and negative thinking based in consequences of use abounds. "As addicts, we turned our will and our lives over many times to a destructive power. Our will and our lives were controlled by drugs."[5] The individual has limited ability to tolerate stressors without the relief gained from the addictive behavior, and must turn to a Higher Power. The familiar is no longer acceptable, self-sufficiency has failed, and a new path must be taken. Yet, this is a very difficult task. One member spoke of the "claw marks" he left on everything he had ever let go of. Turning it over can be considered in two manners: to address a change in cognition by looking to a Higher Power instead of one's selfish motives, and in examining those life events and circumstances that the individual has no control over. This Step is used to develop a new understanding of life related to a Higher Power. This involves not just belief but faith that this Power will take a role in one's affairs. It suggests that individuals can rely on something outside themselves that can be counted on in addressing their daily activities. This is regularly discussed as an act of surrender, and it is a courageous act. This Step results in an attempt to lead one's life based on unfamiliar principles rather than on one's own desires, with faith that life will improve as a result. It is a spiritual practice, absolutely counter to the member's previous routine, a profound change in outlook that places the individuals will in alignment with that of the God of their choosing. "Thy will, not mine, be done."[6]

   "There is only one key, and it is called willingness."[7] To begin this Step, one needs to only become willing, with an expectation that the gains others have made are available to all by following this path. It is a decision in the form of a commitment, which requires repetition to maintain the level of attention necessary to result in a life-changing experience. It requires a decision, not perfection. One is not expected to suddenly lead a perfect existence, but the program always emphasizes progress. "Surrendering to the will of our Higher Power gets easier with daily practice."[8] In making this decision "to turn our will and our lives over to the care of God as we understood Him," one is making a decision to lead a life based on spiritual principle instead of self-interest. It is a decision to get out of the way of one's own progress, to get out of the driver's seat and let a Higher Power take over. Some members have not made conscious personal decisions in their lifetime; this can therefore be seen as a daunting task. Some members have not successfully decided upon an understanding of a God, leaving them unable to proceed with confidence. They are reminded they need only make a decision; they need only be willing to begin this process. This is a choice—it is not forced upon the individual, but it is seen as an essential decision if one is to stay sober. It is extremely important to the newcomer to consider this a decision, as it is all too easy to see it as an impossible task, caught up in the mystery and the difficulty of the concepts it represents.

Step Three uses the concept of a Higher Power established in Step Two but with different terminology. It is the first Step to use the word God, but adds, "as we understood Him." This leaves the individual able to examine a Higher Power in any form they choose, much the same as Step Two. One is not expected to define God but most members do give more consideration to their formulation and understanding of God as they work this Step. Using the term "God" can be troublesome for some people and for those of certain religious backgrounds. People can easily get stuck here and may need to be reminded of the intent of the founders, which was to be inclusive in regard to the spiritual practices of the Steps. The belief confirmed in Step Two is expanded upon in this Step, as people begin to rely on their God to direct their lives and their wills. By defining their own God, people are much more likely to turn things over. Most people are very resistant to giving up control, especially the addict or alcoholic whose life has been run by self-centeredness. To turn over control, to let go, is unnatural, and requires a great deal of faith. This faith comes with time, with the help of others, and with willingness. The understanding of a Higher Power changes over time as people develop, gain experience, and deepen their spiritual practice. The later Steps play a major role in these changes as the result of the spiritual discipline associated with them. The term "God" can be used as a fundamental expression of Higher Power: some describe God as the shortest word or phrase to express the concept of a supreme being; others discuss God as Good Orderly Direction. Some fundamentalist Christians have difficulty with the loose manner in which the term "God" is used by A.A. members, but they, too, have the opportunity to believe according to their personal understanding of God, and they can start their own meetings if necessary.

Step Three reveals the possibility of marked changes that can occur if one chooses to lead a life based on spiritual principles. It requires a willingness to let go of control and take direction, which are very difficult tasks for anyone. Most people have difficulty believing that something outside of themselves will actually care for them in the manner that they wish to be cared for. This is a common topic in meetings about this Step. People discuss their wants versus their needs. The Twelve Step member may want to keep drinking, keep having multiple sexual partners or keep using a certain drug, but by making the "decision" found in Step Three, they realize they actually need to do something much different, something that goes against their own wills. One member shared a story about honesty and the Third Step. He was attempting to discover what this Step meant to him, when he found himself alone in the back room of an outdoor supply store. The store personnel knew and trusted him, so he was allowed to try out a couple of fly rods. He knew more about them than the people working that day, and once alone, began to consider a plan to purchase the very expensive rod by switching price tags with the affordable rod. He was new to recovery and was attempting to turn around a life of dishonesty that included a great deal of theft. He looked over the rods for at least a half hour while struggling with the decision. He wanted the expensive rod, but could not afford it. He also wanted to stay sober and lead a new way of life, based on spiritual principles, in particular, honesty. The "decision" to turn his will and his life over had become personal, directly addressing his desire in a manner that would limit his behavior. Ultimately, he walked out of the store without stealing or changing the tags. He "made a decision" to turn his will and his life over to the care of his God in that moment, a decision that had to be repeated innumerable times in regard to other behaviors to result in lasting change. He chose his spiritual needs over his immediate wants or desires. He chose to follow a spiritual path. Most people in Twelve Step programs will discuss these as life-saving decisions, because to choose "God's will" may keep one sober, while following the negative path, maintaining the dishonesty, can lead to relapse.

The basis of the daily practice of Step Three is in ongoing attempts to examine behavior from an objective stance using thoughts of a Higher Power as a guide in decision-making, rather than individual will. The ability to turn one's will and one's life over is founded in the multiple daily decisions to seek direction from outside oneself, not a single decision. Twelve Step members are expected to compare their own will to God's will and make every attempt to adjust their behavior to what they believe their God would approve of. "Thy will, not mine, be done." It is a true spiritual discipline, a daily, minute-by-minute, adjustment of attitude and behavior, with every decision bringing one closer to a more desirable existence. It is an effort that requires diligent examination of motives, thought patterns, and expectations. Sometimes these decisions require the help of others, to avoid the pitfalls of self-will. Members often discuss decision-making in regard to "God's will" and share their experience with the mystery of turning one's will and one's life over. A young member said he was attempting to work the Third Step during college, early in recovery. He was unable to determine what courses to study on particular days, and believed that his attempt to "turn his will and his life over" should have resulted in answers. When there was no voice, and no lightning strike, he became frustrated and confused. He brought this dilemma to the attention of his sponsor and was told to use his own mind, to make such decisions in a responsible manner. Another member described his ability to convince himself that whatever he wanted had to be God's will. He found this to be a long-standing pattern of self-absorption, and discovered that he had to use a close friend or his sponsor in making such decisions, or he would fool himself into justifying selfish acts. The Step requires the ability to accept direction from outside oneself, whether this is from another person or a Higher Power. It is a Step that results in personal growth due to objective self-examination and an ongoing effort to adjust one's behavior to a higher ideal.

The professional will readily notice how applications of the Third Step resemble cognitive behavioral interventions, with the added element of a Higher Power. This is a practical spirituality that uses self-examination of cognition to address behavioral change. It emphasizes a Higher Power as the ultimate authority, not the individual's ideas, which can be remarkably disturbed secondary to the destructive nature of the addictive process. Although the spiritual aspect of this Step can seem mysterious, breaking down cognitive processes to examine motives in regard to decision-making can be readily described and measured. The individual can recognize when they have stopped to think through a decision with a mind open to outside input, using consideration of God's will, rather than their own immediate desire. This can be discussed as "turning it over," a cognitive intervention, bolstered by the belief that a Higher Power will "restore us to sanity." The faith necessary to Step Three that provides the individual with new strength and conviction is not used in formal cognitive behavioral therapy. This faith, once well established, provides the individual and the therapist with a much more powerful vehicle for change. Using a cognitive behavioral approach is much richer and more effective when the individual understands that they are attempting to do God's will rather than their own. They surrender to a Power greater than themselves, in contrast to formal cognitive behavioral therapy in which one uses cognitive interventions with no sense of an external power or source, relying solely on one's own ability to change thought patterns. This is a difficult and sometimes disturbing thought to the newly recovered alcoholic or addict, whose best thinking resulted in the tragedy of addiction.

The professional can readily discuss the meaning and the difficulties associated with "God as we understood Him." This can be of great benefit to the newcomer as this is a troublesome concept, fraught with bias and misinterpretation. The professional can guide people through some of the personal roadblocks associated with this Step, helping them to develop their own "understanding" of a God. Perfectionism is another problem common to this Step. It is important to look upon this Step as a decision rather than a sudden ability to live up to spiritual goals. Turning it over and surrender are mysterious concepts that lend themselves to the use of examples much more than to frank explanations. Twelve Step members are familiar with the use of examples in the form of stories, which the therapist can use to explain some of the intricacies of this Step. Confusion over "letting go" can be addressed by a standard Twelve Step interpretation; one must release the responsibility for the outcome, not for the effort. Using the concepts of this Step to establish spiritual discipline of examining one's thoughts and behavior with intent to live up to a higher ideal is essential to the entire Twelve Step program, and to good recovery itself. This requires faith, but the daily effort is found in examining thoughts and attempting to change them to match that which one believes a Higher Power would endorse.

Counselors describe distinct characteristics of the person who has begun to actively use this Step. The key appears to be a newfound willingness, in particular a willingness to take direction. They begin to do things foreign to their nature, assessing their motives and acting out of a higher ideal rather than the self-centered perspective of the active alcoholic. These changes are observable and can be used to evaluate and document progress. Although this Step corresponds well with a cognitive behavioral approach, it limits intellectual examination, asking the individual to "turn it over." The professional can play an important role in maintaining the focus on a spiritual approach, and helping the client with an anti-intellectual path to behavioral change. These people have tried to think their way out of this and will continue to do so. It is the role of the therapist to de-emphasize attempts to "figure out" the program, which can undermine a correct focus on the faith necessary to begin a spiritual path and work this simple program.

Inherent in the Third Step is the decision to begin a life-long process devoted to self-examination based on spiritual principles. The basic intent of this Step is to encourage the participant to make a decision to live a new way of life. This can evolve into a remarkable change in perspective and conduct, in which destructive self-centeredness is replaced by an ability to reach out for help and guidance from a Higher Power. The individual further defines his or her understanding of God, and begins to rely on a God that takes a role in daily affairs. This role is found in the daily decision-making to live by a higher ideal, and in the corresponding miracles that occur and strengthen one's faith. This Step is a commitment to a spiritual path that places the individual's will subordinate to "God's will," with the expectation that one is capable of leading a profoundly better life. It is the essence of this spiritual program.

The Third Step prayer from *Alcoholics Anonymous*:

God, I offer myself to Thee—to build with me and do with me as thou wilt. Relieve me of the bondage of self, that I may better do Thy will. Take away my difficulties, that victory over them may bear witness to those I would help of Thy Power, Thy Love, and Thy Way of Life. May I do Thy will always.[9]

REFERENCES

1. *The Twelve Steps and Twelve Traditions* (New York: Alcoholics Anonymous World Services, Inc., 1988) p. 34.
2. *The Twelve Steps and Twelve Traditions* (New York: Alcoholics Anonymous World Services, Inc., 1988) pp. 34–35.
3. *Alcoholics Anonymous, 3rd Ed.* (New York: A.A. World Services, Inc., 1976) p. 62.
4. *Alcoholics Anonymous, 3rd Ed.* (New York: A.A. World Services, Inc., 1976) p. 60.
5. *Narcotics Anonymous, 5th Ed.* (Van Nuys, CA: N.A. World Services, Inc., 1988) p. 24.

6. *The Twelve Steps and Twelve Traditions* (New York: Alcoholics Anonymous World Services, Inc., 1988) p. 103.

7. *The Twelve Steps and Twelve Traditions* (New York: Alcoholics Anonymous World Services, Inc., 1988), p. 34.

8. *Narcotics Anonymous, 5th Ed.* (Van Nuys, CA: N.A. World Services, Inc., 1988), p. 25.

9. *Alcoholics Anonymous, 3rd Ed.* (New York: A.A. World Services, Inc., 1976) p. 63.

Chapter Eight

Steps Four and Five

"Made a searching and fearless moral inventory of ourselves."
"Admitted to God, to ourselves, and to another human being, the exact nature of our wrongs."

These two Steps serve as a profound inquiry into one's life, based on actual behavior, initiated with an inventory, and completed by expressing wrongdoing "to God, to ourselves, and to another human being." The Fourth and Fifth Steps are distinct tasks, but intrinsically linked as a rite of passage which requires an even greater depth of honesty than considered to this point. The individual has completed the first three Steps (admitting to a problem, developing the foundation of belief in a Higher Power, and deciding to live by spiritual principles) in preparation for self-examination that is unusual to most people's experience. These may be the two most discussed Steps of the program, yet the most frequently skipped or neglected due to the intense level of examination and exposure that is required. These Steps are not new concepts or ideas for the individual to contemplate; they are action Steps that directly engage denial and self-deception, contributing remarkably to self-acceptance. One cannot correct or change behavior without first knowing what problems exist. These two Steps initiate a healing process that begins to address deep-seated guilt and shame, releasing people from their past mistakes. A basic premise of Twelve Step programs is that one is likely to return to addictive behavior if one does not address the past, expose one's secrets, and begin this healing process. It is one thing to think about life change, growth, and spirituality, and quite another to write a personal moral inventory and then admit wrongs to someone else. "The purpose of a searching and fearless moral inventory is to sort through the confusion and contradiction of our lives, so that we can find out who we really are. We are starting a new way of life and need to be rid of the burdens and traps that controlled us and prevented our growth."[1]

Step 4: "Made a searching and fearless moral inventory of ourselves."

Step 4 is a very difficult undertaking for any individual. One is asked to take a "searching and fearless" look at oneself, frankly examining the behavior that had been avoided through denial and self-deception. "Step Four is our vigorous and painstaking effort to discover what these liabilities in each of us have been, and are. We want to find exactly how, when and where our natural desires have warped us. ... By discovering what our emotional deformities are, we can move toward their correction. Without a willing and persistent effort to do this, there can be little sobriety or contentment for us. Without a searching and fearless inventory, most of us found that the faith which really works in daily living is still out of reach."[2] No definition of "moral inventory" exists in Twelve Step literature; the moral decisions described in this undertaking are up to the individual. It is believed that each of us has a solid sense of right and wrong, and can examine our own behavior justly. Once again the individual is held accountable and responsible for the fulfillment of a difficult task, without specific written instruction, with an expectation that proper motivation will result in an appropriate effort and provide the necessary experience. These are suggested Steps, up to the individual to perform at the level they choose. The results are dependent upon the individual's effort, but experience reveals great yields from proper execution. Peers and sponsors are available for advice and direction in regard to this "personal house cleaning."[3]

The individual is to be as honest and thorough as possible; no one can remember every detail, but the expectation is to fully examine one's life, not just the addictive behavior and its consequences. Honest self-examination of this type is unnatural, and places the individual in direct conflict with denial and self-deception, the very traits that have fostered the problems that are to be considered. This can scare off many people who are not ready for this level of self-examination and honesty. This is a very painful process for the person who has worked to avoid looking at themselves and the consequences of their behavior. People are advised to be complete, to write down in particular the life experiences they are least likely to tell another, those events one does not even want to revisit or think about. Dick M. describes these as "the shadow at the bottom of the bucket." The essence of this discipline is to get out the most shameful events of one's life, to get it on paper, and begin to relieve the power that these dark secrets hold. The level of willingness to do this is associated with the success of the endeavor.

This is to be a true inventory; it should document both attributes and liabilities. When a business does an inventory, it includes that which has been lost, damaged and stolen, as well as what is left in stock, what has been sold, and how much money has been made. People in early recovery often focus on the negative, neglecting assets that are essential to a thorough examination of self. The individual needs to witness the foundation of positive attributes upon which to build a new life. The examination of assets also reveals values that may have appeared lost due to the addictive lifestyle. Recognition of these latent attributes can help in the reestablishment of a life based solidly on spiritual values.

The inventory is to be used to examine specific incidents as well as patterns of behavior. Major life events are easy to recall and address, but a pattern of dishonesty or manipulation in relationships requires a different type of examination. It is useful for the individual to document numerous incidents of a similar type or under a specific topic. This can reveal unrecognized links and patterns that become meaningful only when placed on paper. The Fourth Step is set up to develop self-awareness and self-knowledge. The emphasis is on "ourselves"—no one else. The proper use of this Step reveals how the individual has blamed other people and circumstance when the real problem lies within. With repetitive examples and details from varied arenas, one begins to piece together a reasonable mosaic of one's life. As this is revealed, the individual has the choice to continue to grow and change or turn one's back on this newfound awareness.

The Fourth Step is intended to be a written inventory. It is not adequate to do it by memory, in one's head, which is a common mistake. It requires an objective examination of behavior, not available to the individual if it is unwritten. One can continue to fool oneself with denial and other forms of self-deception, if it is not addressed outside of memory. Thoughts must be organized to be written, which helps in examining the behavioral patterns that are a key to this Step. It is much more striking to the individual to see his or her inventory on paper, than it is to think it through again.

It is important to use a format of some sort to complete Step Four. The Big Book provides an example of a Fourth Step that is regularly used. This inventory emphasizes examination of resentment, fear, and sex. Other pamphlets and workbooks have been written to guide people through a Fourth Step inventory. These tend to be more involved than the Big Book, examining broader, more diverse aspects of life. They also use more specific instructions, which can be of help to the newcomer. The recommendation to be "searching and fearless," honest and thorough, remains the same independent of the resource used. One is expected to use specific examples of life events. It is to be a detailed undertaking. I recommend that people examine a few of these methods to find one that fits for them. A sponsor can be of help in this regard.

It is beneficial to schedule the Fourth Step, specifying a time for completion. This is an extremely important but difficult Step. It is very easy to procrastinate because of the nature of the task. It is best to initiate the inventory and complete it without delay. Some of the wounds that are opened and exposed can be extremely painful, and need to be addressed and contained, not left to haunt the individual. In spite of the pain and difficulty involved, this healing process is a definitive task that needs to be attended to. Often people will postpone or avoid this Step because they get ahead of themselves thinking about the Fifth Step, worrying that someone else will learn so much about them, and that they will expose their darkest secrets to another human being. This is not uncommon and must be guarded against. To do a legitimate inventory requires maintaining focus on the task at hand, taking an honest look at oneself and putting the whole story on paper.

"By now the newcomer has probably arrived at the following conclusions: that his character defects, representing instincts gone astray, have been the primary cause of his drinking and his failure at life, that unless he is now willing to work hard at the elimination of the worst of these defects, both sobriety and peace of mind will still elude him; that all the faulty foundation of his life will have to be torn out and built anew on bedrock."[4] By directly examining behavior in a manner that limits denial and self-deception, one can get an accurate look at oneself and begin to get to know oneself without the veil of self-interest. This Step allows one to actually witness the changes undergone during the active addiction and set sights on a new life. The individual becomes more accountable for his or her own behavior, and much less likely to blame others and circumstances. "Once we have a complete willingness to take inventory, and exert ourselves to do the job thoroughly, a wonderful light falls upon this foggy scene. As we persist, a brand new kind of confidence is born, and the sense of relief at finally facing ourselves is indescribable. These are the fruits of Step Four."[4]

This Step begins the process of dealing with shame and guilt in an active, purposeful manner. Documenting the very acts that resulted in the ongoing shame is a powerful tool in gaining self-forgiveness. It is in exposing these acts to the light of day that allows the individual to gain a new self-perspective, rather than maintaining the "secrets that keep us sick." Self-acceptance and a sense of humility begin to occur replacing the lonely existence of shame. People begin to gain enjoyment in their lives as problems are addressed and they gain relief from the shame and guilt associated with their past behavior. "We must be done with the past, not cling to it. We want to look our past in the face, see it for what it really was and release it so we can live today."[5]

"Honest self-assessment is one of the keys to our new way of life."[1] The examination of assets establishes a baseline from which to build, while documenting frailties, faults, and defects establishes direction for change. The individual is given a choice, through self-examination, to begin the difficult process of change with the raw material at hand, the reality of one's behavior. This Step can provide the necessary motivation to continue these Steps and address repetitive cycles of negative behavior. Nonetheless this Step is limited in one respect: self-examination can suffer from the very problems it attempts to expose; more needs to be done. "It is our experience that no matter how searching and thorough, no inventory is of any lasting effect unless it is promptly followed by an equally thorough Fifth Step."[6]

Step 5: "Admitted to God, to ourselves, and to another human being, the exact nature of our wrongs." ....

"All of A.A.'s Twelve Steps ask us to go contrary to our natural desires ... they all deflate our egos. When it comes to ego deflation, few steps are harder to take than Five. But scarcely any step is more necessary to long-time sobriety and peace of mind than this one."[7] People discuss "doing a Fifth Step," with pride and reverence. It is a courageous act that requires a level of self-disclosure seldom considered and often feared. Willingness to be fully exposed and to take direction are required. In essence, one is to describe the "wrongs" documented in their Fourth Step, their moral inventory with all their secrets, "to God, to ourselves, and to another human being." This is a monumental task for anyone, but it is completely unnatural to the addict or alcoholic. This Step involves a greater level of risk, related to the fear of exposure, than any other Step. It can result in the release of a tremendous burden, a true catharsis, which contributes to the metamorphosis

of the sincere individual. Not only does one experience "ego deflation," one begins to gain an understanding of true humility.
"Another great dividend we may expect from confiding our defects
to another human being is humility—a word often misunderstood.
To those who have made progress in A.A., it amounts to a clear
recognition of what and who we really are, followed by a sincere
attempt to become what we could be. Therefore, our first practical
move toward humility must consist of recognizing our deficien-
cies."[8] The Fifth Step is concerned with "the exact nature of our
wrongs," the spirit of our transgressions, or the "spiritlessness"
of how one is living. It does not just ask that one recite the incidents,
but that one look beyond the behavior into the "nature" of what it
is to be human, and "not-God." This Step is truly a rite of passage,
necessary to a new life based on spiritual principles. It requires
and defines a new level of honesty for the individual. Some people
do not achieve the goal, as they are unable to fully expose themselves, hoping to avoid certain events, details, or truths about
themselves. "They took inventory all right, but hung on to some of
the worst items in stock. They thought they had lost their egoism
and fear, they only thought they had humbled themselves. But
they had not learned enough of humility, fearlessness, and honesty, in the sense we find necessary, until they told someone else
all their life story."[9]

The distinction between the Fourth and Fifth Steps is vital to
the understanding and proper execution of these Steps. "We have
admitted certain defects; we have ascertained in a rough way
what the trouble is; we have put our finger on the weak items in
our personal inventory. Now these are about to be cast out. This is
perhaps difficult—especially discussing our defects with another
person. We think we have done well enough in admitting these
things to ourselves. There is doubt about that. In actual practice,
we usually find a solitary self-appraisal insufficient."[10] "Hence it
was most evident that a solitary self-appraisal, and the admission
of our defects based upon that alone would not be nearly enough.
We would have to have outside help if we were surely to know and
admit the truth about ourselves—the help of God and another
human being. Only by discussing ourselves, holding back nothing,

only by being willing to take advice and accept direction could we set foot on the road to straight thinking, solid honesty, and genuine humility."[11] These quotes reveal the intended difference between the two Steps and some of the expectations the originators had in mind. These Steps are linked directly to Oxford Group practices of confession and sharing. In the Fourth Step the individual fully documents their life in the form of a "moral inventory"; in the Fifth Step they expose themselves.

The Fifth Step should be completed shortly after one has accomplished the Fourth Step. With "solitary self-appraisal insufficient" one moves outside of oneself to complete the Fifth Step and expel the secrets, moving beyond documentation of shameful, guilt-ridden acts into a position of healing with the help of a Higher Power and the acceptance of another human being. One must choose the person to work with wisely, due to the type of information that is to be discussed and in order to minimize some of the fear and anxiety related to the act. Many people use a sponsor, which can work out very well in sharing details of one's life and establishing an honest, open relationship. Clergy are often chosen due to the nature of the Step, and they are obligated to secrecy. Physicians and therapists are also asked to complete this Step with people. It is important for the professional to have a solid working knowledge of this Step especially if providing this service for someone. The receiver of the Fifth Step must maintain a contemplative, accepting stance. This is an act of healing for the individual, who is reticent, scared, and unsure of following through with it. The other "human being" must be able to acknowledge the depth of sharing, and engage in the process without surprise, judgment, or blame. It is up to the other "human being" to listen intently and then enter into a dialogue about the way in which the Step was done, review some of the more important aspects of the experience, provide feedback about some behaviors and patterns that may not have been obvious to the person, and address the benefits of the Step. It is also important to note a poor quality Fifth Step, to ask for a more compete job, or to suggest that the individual start over or get more honest.

It is best to complete the Fifth Step in a single session, with no interruptions. The emphasis is on recounting one's life, releasing the "wrongs," and exposing oneself. Some people will avoid certain life events or topics, limiting their disclosure as they are unable to fully address themselves. Others will exaggerate—usually positive attributes—or they will attempt to gloss over the negative in hopes that they would not have to fully reveal themselves. It is recommended that the individual "get it all out"; holding back certain life events maintains secrets, which will often continue to haunt the person and can result in relapse. The manner in which one completes this task, in particular the depth of honest self-disclosure, will reveal the individual's commitment to their growth and recovery.

After completion of the Fifth Step most people contemplate their accomplishment in quiet self-reflection. This is an opportunity to take in the experience in a bit more objective manner and savor the feeling of relief that is usually associated with this Step. People often describe feeling as if a great weight has been lifted, and find themselves free of some of the secrets that they have been carrying. Twelve Step literature does not address the written account of the Fourth Step or whatever notes are used in doing a Fifth Step. Thoughts about this differ, but in general, people believe that maintaining the written account is not helpful and can be dangerous. This Step is about releasing demons, so keeping the account goes against this concept, and can be another way of hanging onto the negative events of one's past. It is also risky to keep a document of one's past transgressions available for others to come upon and read. I suggest people use a formal ritual, to bury or burn the written record, while reflecting on release of the past. This tends to enhance the experience, and destroys the evidence.

Step Five diminishes self-delusion and denial in a sweeping manner, leaving the individual on the verge of a marked life change. For the sincere, this Step provides freedom from the past, allowing one to begin a new way of life that is no longer influenced by the negative power of the addiction and its consequences. Shame and guilt are specifically addressed, continuing the process of releasing the individual from their influence. This is done in a manner that holds the person accountable for past misdeeds while promoting this new life, thus changing behavior in a manner that allows for the resolution of the shame and guilt, not just by thinking that it is so, but by behavioral change.

Revealing oneself to someone else and a Higher Power results in a marked advance in self-acceptance and the beginning of self-forgiveness. "This vital step was also the means by which we began to get the feeling that we could be forgiven, no matter what we had thought or done."[8] The experience of the Fifth Step, in which one shares "the shadow at the bottom of the bucket" and is accepted by "another human being" promotes self-acceptance. Individuals are sharing information that they never wanted anyone else to know about their lives and thoughts, and the other person does not lecture them or leave the room in shock. They experience acceptance, a sense of their own humanity, and the essence of humility. They have been incredibly honest about themselves in a manner that will continue to promote a life in which the individual is more real and more honest with others. This new-found level of acceptance ensures a degree of self-forgiveness that has eluded the individual during active addiction. As the individual works the rest of the Steps and incorporates this program into daily life, they experience a freedom from the past that they did not believe possible, and slowly forgive themselves for the way of life they once led.

This Step allows the individual to move forward without having to carry the enormous load of past problems. It provides the foundation and direction for a new, spiritually based life. It relieves some of the shame, guilt, and fear related to behavior and secrets that has kept the individual separate from others and constantly feeling "less than." The Fifth Step provides a positive experience with humility as the result of a conscious review of actual behavior and an examination of how one has lived while pursuing self-interest above all else. After this Step, the person on a spiritual path can share themselves more easily and fully with others having been freed of the limiting effects of self-deception and dishonesty. "We pocket our pride and go to it, illuminating every twist of character, every dark cranny of the past. Once we have taken this step, withholding nothing, we are delighted. We can look the world in the eye. We can be alone at perfect peace and ease. Our fears fall from us. We begin to feel the nearness of our Creator. We may have had certain spiritual beliefs, but now we begin to have a spiritual experience. That feeling that the drink problem has disappeared will often come strongly. We feel we are on the Broad Highway, walking hand in hand with the Spirit of the Universe."[12]

The professional needs a solid understanding of the remarkable implications of these two Steps. They are grounded by the necessity to come clean, fully examining and then exposing oneself, in order to continue to advance on a spiritual path. These Steps emphasize accountability for one's actions in order to establish a foundation for growth. The level of honesty required is once again a formidable task for most people, and may not make sense to the therapist, but is essential to these Steps. The professional should encourage the full disclosure, "searching and fearless" as described by the Twelve Step literature, but must be clear that this is a personal examination of one's behavior, not other people's problems or behaviors. It can be helpful for the professional to encourage completion of these Steps, especially when fear or procrastination prevent this. Direction about the type of Fourth Step to do, in particular the type of guide to use, can be beneficial. The professional can advise the person doing a Fourth Step about the manner in which they are proceeding; if it is inadequate, limited and less than honest, one can direct them to improve. On the other hand some people will become obsessive and perfectionist, requiring limits and boundaries. While some people will be paralyzed by fear, others will be paralyzed by perfection, and the professional can provide appropriate direction. If you are chosen to hear a Fifth Step it is important to fully understand your role. The request suggests a marked degree of trust in the professional, and entails a long session of intimate details about the individual. It is recommended that the Fifth Step be accomplished in a single session. It is important to be accepting and nonjudgmental. It is not the usual role of a therapist—to hear a Fifth Step, the clinician must listen, provide appropriate feedback as it relates to the information divulged, and discuss the benefits of the experience, especially as they relate to leading a spiritual life. The discussion should also attend to the ongoing task of resolving shame and guilt, as well as attending to self-acceptance and self-forgiveness. Following such a procedure honors the Step, not the professional's orientation. It is not necessary to agree to hear a Fifth Step if you do not feel comfortable doing so, but it can be an inspiring experience for the listener as well as the person working the Step.

REFERENCES

1. *Narcotics Anonymous, 5th Ed.* (Van Nuys, CA: N.A. World Services, Inc., 1988) p. 26.
2. *The Twelve Steps and Twelve Traditions* (New York: Alcoholics Anonymous World Services, Inc., 1988) p. 44.
3. *Alcoholics Anonymous, 3rd Ed.* (New York: A.A. World Services, Inc., 1976) p. 63.
4. *The Twelve Steps and Twelve Traditions* (New York: Alcoholics Anonymous World Services, Inc., 1988) p. 51.
5. *Narcotics Anonymous, 5th Ed.* (Van Nuys, CA: N.A. World Services, Inc., 1988) p. 27.
6. *Narcotics Anonymous, 5th Ed.* (Van Nuys, CA: N.A. World Services, Inc., 1988) p. 29
7. *The Twelve Steps and Twelve Traditions* (New York: Alcoholics Anonymous World Services, Inc., 1988) p. 56.
8. *The Twelve Steps and Twelve Traditions* (New York: Alcoholics Anonymous World Services, Inc., 1988) p. 59.
9. *The Twelve Steps and Twelve Traditions* (New York: Alcoholics Anonymous World Services, Inc., 1988) p. 73.
10. *The Twelve Steps and Twelve Traditions* (New York: Alcoholics Anonymous World Services, Inc., 1988) p. 72.
11. *The Twelve Steps and Twelve Traditions* (New York: Alcoholics Anonymous World Services, Inc., 1988) p. 60.
12. *Alcoholics Anonymous, 3rd Ed.* (New York: A.A. World Services, Inc., 1976) p. 75.

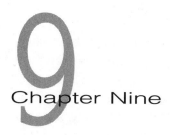

Chapter Nine

Steps Six and Seven

"Were entirely ready to have God remove all these defects of character."
"Humbly asked Him to remove our shortcomings."

These two Steps embody the essence of self-change. The first five Steps have established the main problem, described a spiritual solution, and documented associated problems and difficulties. These two Steps ask the individual to decide if he or she wants to continue to change and offer a strategy to do so, one which requires a new level of faith and trust. This is consistent with any spiritual path; individuals must begin to face themselves and decide if they want to pursue a more desirable existence based upon spiritual principles. These Steps move well beyond the initial goal of abstinence and suggest that much more work is to be done, and much more is to be gained. This provides hope as most people in recovery recognize that abstinence, in and of itself, is not enough. They know they must change in a variety of ways, and it is even clearer to them, once clean and sober, that life could be pretty miserable if they continued to live in the manner in which they have been accustomed, with or without drugs and alcohol. These Steps represent a lifetime of effort—there are no quick fixes. They provide the framework for continued growth and development. The Narcotics Anonymous (N.A.) text describes this very well: "This is our road to spiritual growth. We change every day. We gradually and carefully pull ourselves out of the isolation and loneliness of addiction and into the mainstream of life."[1]

These are overlooked Steps that offer opportunities for significant personal growth. The *Alcoholics Anonymous* text devotes only a single paragraph to each. A Hazelden pamphlet about Steps 6 and 7 is entitled "The Forgotten Steps." They are referred to as the "nodders" around Twelve Step meetings, suggesting that people nod with acknowledgment when they are discussed but fail to rigorously work these Steps and as a result have little to share of their experience with them. Those who do work these two Steps gain tremendously, and are able to address faults and shortcomings in a manner that requires another act of surrender to a Higher Power. These Steps are built upon the foundation established in the first three Steps, which reveal a Higher Power that takes an active role in one's daily life. The requirements are simple: become ready, and then ask for help.

These two Steps suggest attention is paid to "defects of character" and "shortcomings." There is no frank definition of what is meant by these two terms. The A.A. literature refers to lists developed from the Fifth Step, and there are some examples provided. "Character defects or shortcomings are those things that cause pain and misery all of our lives."[2] "Since most of us have been born with an abundance of natural desires it is not strange that we often let these far exceed their intended purpose. When they drive us blindly, or we willfully demand that they supply us with more satisfactions or pleasures than are possible or due us, that is the point at which we depart from the degree of perfection that God wishes for us here on earth. That is the measure of our character defects, or, if you wish, of our sins."[3] The inventory done in the Fourth Step, and further self-examination specific to the Fifth Step readily reveal enough information for the individual to develop an understanding, if not a list, of "defects" and "shortcomings."

Step Six: "Were entirely ready to have God remove all these defects of character."

The A.A. text devotes only this statement to the Sixth Step: "Is our work solid so far? Are the stones properly in place? Have we skimped on the cement put into the foundation? ... If we can answer to our satisfaction, we then look at Step Six. We have emphasized willingness as being indispensable. Are we now ready to have God remove from us all the things that we have admitted are objectionable? Can He now take them all—every one? If we still cling to something we will not let go, we ask God to help us be willing."[4] Step Six is a spiritual exercise of preparation for personal growth. While on a spiritual path, involved in personal growth, one will inevitably come to a point in which there is recognition of the need to change specific characteristics. Often this recognition is the result of pain. This pain is secondary to living with defects of character that get in the way of reaching one's potential. Some of this is identifiable while using drugs and alcohol, but most comes into focus only after the person has entered into recovery as a result of working these Steps with attention to spiritual growth. At this point the person on such a path has a decision to make: do I want to change, to continue to grow, to fully develop my potential and myself? This Step can be considered a way of examining one's desires, especially those that are out of control or excessive, in order to reign in the ego and establish new goals based on spiritual principles.

The Sixth Step requires willingness, to be "entirely ready" to change. It should be done right after Step Five when shortcomings are readily recognized and the individual is highly motivated for change. Becoming "entirely ready" to change is not an easy task. *Drop the Rock*, a book about Steps 6 and 7, suggests four reasons why people have difficulty being ready: (1) a conscious decision not to change, or give up, a particular defect; (2) blaming defects on others, or on circumstances—an inability to recognize one's role; (3) rationalizing the problems away—they are not that bad, nor do they need to be changed; (4) denial, the person is unaware of the problem.[5] Fear can also be an issue that prevents people from working this Step. Fear that they cannot do it well enough, fear that they cannot change, and fear that they are unworthy of change. Many people have started this Step only to hesitate when faced with a "defect" they believe they cannot do anything about or one that they do not want to address, often giving up on the whole task, with thoughts that they must be perfect. There is also a tendency to enjoy some of our defects, which limits the ability to change them. "What we must realize is that we exult in some of our defects. We really love them."[6] This Step emphasizes readiness, in the form of willingness, not a sudden change implying sainthood or perfectionism. The individual is being asked to wholeheartedly and willingly focus on living a better life based on spiritual principles. "This is a Step of willingness. Willingness is the spiritual principle of Step Six."[2]

The Step appears to suggest a degree of perfection that can be frightening to the initiate. As mentioned, the emphasis is on willingness, not perfection, but the Step uses the words "entirely" and "all," leaving the individual faced with a daunting task. Many people have stopped work on this Step due to the inability to accomplish it in a perfect manner. They take an all-or-nothing approach, and stop when they recognize something they do not want to be rid of. This Step asks the individual to prepare for a Higher Power to do something; it does not ask individuals to completely relieve themselves of all their defects. Becoming ready is the task at hand, and it is fraught with enough difficulty. "How many of us have this degree of readiness? In an absolute sense practically nobody has it. The best we can do, with all the honesty we can summon, is to try to have it. Even then the best of us will discover to our dismay that there is always a sticking point, a point at which we say, 'No, I cannot give this up yet.' And we shall tread on an even more dangerous ground when we cry, 'This I will never give up.' "[7] The tendency is to view the Step as impossible, difficult to grasp, almost ethereal. Since it is not well understood, and involves terminology that suggests perfection, people easily balk, rather than pursuing a better understanding of the task. This Step is about "progress rather than ... perfection."[8] "So Step Six— 'were entirely ready to have God remove these defects of character'—is A.A.'s way of stating the best possible attitude one can take in order to make a beginning on this lifetime job. This does not mean that we expect all our character defects to be lifted out of us as the drive to drink was. A few of them may be, but with most of them we shall have to be content with patient improvement."[9] In spite of the pitfalls of perfectionism associated with this Step, the wording places the individual in a position of self-examination with lofty goals. "We shall need to raise our eyes toward perfection, and be ready to walk in that direction."[10] To correctly work this Step the individual must be willing to glance at perfection and work toward it, with the knowledge that humans can only seek to be God-like, but will never reach this goal. It is difficult to maintain an appropriate, balanced stance in regard to this Step, and the individual may need a great deal of assistance which can be provided by a professional. It is not easy to aim at perfection while accepting human limitations. Some do not even want to try, while others will rationalize a level of "perfection" that allows them to live as they please. It can be very helpful to ask the individual if they are "entirely willing" to lead a spiritual life, or "entirely willing" to lead the life of their own choosing, to determine their understanding of this quandary, and their stance.

Step Six also states that the individual must be ready "to have God remove these defects of character." Many people perceive this inaccurately, as if they have to be ready to expel these "defects of character" themselves, that it is their action that results in the changes. This is not intended. The Step is about preparation, willingness, and faith. This Step is the beginning of a journey—it suggests a deeper level of spiritual belief and understanding, taking the individual past the healing acts directed toward the addictive behavior, to address personal growth. This type of attention to self, an attempt to invoke spiritual forces to directly address individual characteristics, is a Step that requires a tremendous degree of faith. One prepares, or becomes "entirely ready" in two ways: first, by recognition of the defects to be addressed; and second, by developing the faith that a Higher Power will "remove" them. Being ready is an act of faith, and engages the person in the task, placing him or her on a path that requires ongoing attention to personal growth. To be ready to have all one's defects removed by a Higher Power is a tremendously difficult stance to take in one's life. It suggests a willingness to examine all one's thoughts and behaviors, with a higher calling, from a spiritual perspective, and with the belief that the process of recovery will unfold in such a way that the proper changes will be attended to by that Higher Power. This does not absolve the individual of responsibility, however; in fact, it is in the readiness that the Steps main function is stated and experienced. According to people who have really worked this Step, the changes occur "in God's time." Being ready is essential to the growth of the individual but does not mean that the defects are suddenly gone. This degree of willingness is another act of surrender. Individuals take full account of themselves and make a decision to live a life based on spiritual discipline, attempting to improve upon every possible aspect of themselves by looking to a Higher Power for the capacity to experience life in an entirely different manner.

This Step is a life-time undertaking. There is no true completion; it is an ongoing effort to establish and maintain willingness and faith, which can result in continued growth and development. The individual attempts to maintain readiness rather than any sort of perfectionist assumption that they have completed the task. The readiness and faith will wax and wane over time, so diligence is needed. Often this Step will require minute-by-minute attention, for willingness to change will be required on a regular basis specific to life events. The readiness established in Step Six is necessary before moving on to Step Seven.

Step Seven: "Humbly asked Him to remove our shortcomings."

The *Alcoholics Anonymous* text devotes a single paragraph in the form of a prayer to the Seventh Step. "When we are ready we say something like this: 'My Creator I am now willing that you should have all of me, good and bad. I pray that you now remove from me every single defect of character that stands in the way of my usefulness to you and my fellows. Grant me strength, as I go out from here, to do your bidding. Amen.' We have then completed Step Seven."[11]

Twelve Steps and Twelve Traditions emphasizes humility as the key to Step Seven. Humility is a very difficult concept for many people. Our culture, which extols "rugged individualism," does not lend itself to recognizing need and requesting help. The rigid nature of many alcoholics and addicts, who have relied entirely on themselves to this point, leaves them hesitant to accept that a Higher Power could do anything about their "shortcomings," even after the remarkable experience of the prior Steps that has resulted in abstinence based on this belief. The establishment of sobriety is often an act of desperation, easing the route to faith; like any "fox hole" belief, someone in dire straits finds that he or she can pray, after all. This Step confirms that individuals on a spiritual path continue to require specific guidance to effectively address their "shortcomings," that they cannot do this by themselves any more than they could stop drinking or using by themselves. The Twelve Steps establish humility as a positive trait, essential to the recovery process. "Indeed, the attainment of greater humility is the foundation of each of A.A.'s Twelve Steps. For without some degree of humility, no alcoholic can stay sober at all. Nearly all A.A.'s have found, too, that unless they develop much more of this precious quality than may be required just for sobriety, they still haven't much chance of becoming truly happy."[12]

Humility allows the individual to recognize limits, and seek help from a Higher Power, allowing the process of positive change to take shape. This Step is the result of belief that relying on a Higher Power rather than on our finite selves can alter personal characteristics. This is a huge undertaking. Not only do individuals have to admit the need to continue to grow and change, they must rely on a mystical, spiritual solution. The recognition that one is "not-God" is essential to the establishment of humility. By working these Steps individuals are able to glimpse the truth about themselves, then ask for help from a Higher Power to shape their lives. This is not the usual route to behavioral or attitudinal change that we support in this culture, nor do most of our psychotherapies support such an approach. This is a spiritual solution, requiring acceptance, faith, and surrender; only by such a path can humility be understood and established. "As long as we placed self-reliance first, a genuine reliance upon a Higher Power was out of the question. That basic ingredient of all humility, a desire to seek and do God's will, was missing."[13]

"For those who have made progress in the program, humility is simply a clear recognition of what and who they are."[14] Humility, as used in Twelve Step programs, is not about humiliation or groveling. It is considered an essential trait based on modesty and unpretentiousness that is born of the marked tragedy people have endured to find themselves in the position of having to work a spiritual program of recovery. The calamity of addiction undermines even the most confident among them. As mentioned, to reestablish a positive sense of self, individuals must turn to a Higher Power, and in so doing admit to the limitations of being human. To establish a faith that one will be healed is essential to initial abstinence, but that is only the beginning of the life-changing efforts summarized in the Twelve Steps. The Seventh Step substantiates the role of humility, which requires both acceptance of self and reliance on a Higher Power. "Everywhere we looked we saw failure and misery transformed by humility into priceless assets. We heard story after story of how humility had brought strength out of weakness."[15]

Some people describe this as the "character building" Step. They are referring to the emphasis on making as much as one can out of life, with the help of a Higher Power. This Step assumes that faith has been established, and that the individual on a spiritual path is willing to continuously work toward a higher level of human experience. This means ongoing attempts to change that which one identifies as problematic. "We had lacked the perspective to see that character-building and spiritual values had to come first, and that material satisfactions were not the purpose of living."[16] This quote reveals the essence of this Step. Most addicts and alcoholics are caught up in self-indulgence in addition to the addiction itself. Negative characteristics that have surfaced during self-examination need to be addressed in a formal manner. This Step goes beyond the obvious and most problematic of the "defects" to suggest ongoing self-improvement consistent with active attention to spiritual values. When people enter a program designed to help them refrain from addictive behavior, they do not expect to find themselves faced with the expectations of the Sixth and Seventh Steps. "Seldom did we look at character-building as something desirable in itself, something we would like to strive for whether our instinctual needs were met or not. We never thought of making honesty, tolerance, and true love of man and God the daily basis of living."[13]

The Seventh Step is a request for help, made to a Higher Power. It engages the individual in an attempt to seek help, rather than seeking another behavioral strategy to change themselves, requiring a great deal of faith that this Power will actually work in their daily lives. It is an act of surrender, much like the Third Step, as the individual is directed to ask to have the shortcomings removed, relying on something outside of him or herself for the life-changing experiences found in the Promises (see pages 41–42). One prepares for this spiritual act in the Sixth Step, and then begins the process of change by making this request. Once again an act of surrender empowers the individual to act with the belief that a Higher Power is working in one's daily life, giving the individual the ability to live differently, to begin the process of change, in any moment. This type of surrender can result in frank behavioral change as the individual, in an act of faith, begins to examine a new way of being.

This Step results in a natural transformation, but the faith and surrender necessary for this are not easy to come by, let alone sustain, so a consistent effort is required. The effort, or the act of working this Step, is in the asking. This is not a Step that can be accomplished by *thinking* about change; it is necessary to ask for help. To approach a Higher Power with the belief necessary to adequately work this Step is considered necessary to experience the desired changes. Some people discuss the point at which they surrendered, when they realized that they could no longer make headway by avoiding some of their "shortcomings" or by trying to *make* themselves different. They talk of getting on their knees and asking for help, sometimes out of desperation, to rid themselves of the behaviors that continue to limit them in recovery. People discuss the freedom provided in this Step, the potential it brings to their lives and their relationships, after they surrender themselves to their Higher Power with the belief that they will be changed. This all hinges on the establishment of humility. "The whole emphasis of Step Seven is on humility. It is really saying to us that we now ought to be willing to try humility in seeking the removal of our shortcomings, just as we did when we admitted that we were powerless over alcohol, and came to believe that a Power greater than ourselves could restore us to sanity. If that degree of humility could enable us to find the grace by which such a deadly obsession could be banished, then there must be hope of the same result respecting any other problem we could possibly have."[17]

A member of A.A. described his experience with the Sixth and Seventh Steps as they related to his problems with honesty. As he entered early recovery he was told repeatedly that this is an honesty program, but he was a habitual liar. He wanted to be honest, but continued to lie on a daily basis. His lying had essentially become a way of life, and he was unable to stop even though he was trying. It was to the point that the first thing out of his mouth was usually a lie, which became even more pronounced as he completed his Fifth Step. The lying seemed designed to allow him to feel better about himself, because he did not have to describe how he really felt, but it actually did the opposite. He felt increasingly ashamed that he was lying, and it left him unable to get close to anyone. As he realized this he tried even harder to stop lying but nothing changed. He was attending A.A. meetings regularly, working with a sponsor, and had been sober for several months. He began to examine the Sixth Step and found that he had not yet even thought in the terms described by the Step. He thought he had to eliminate the lying, and had not considered the possibility that a Higher Power could remove this defect. He began to examine whether or not he was entirely ready for this, as he still used the lies to cover up his behavior and sometimes his real thoughts that he did not want to expose to others. Telling the truth would also force him to state an honest opinion, rather than always agreeing with others. The ramifications went well beyond his initial thoughts about quitting lying due to the pain it was causing in his life. He considered his decision in the Third Step, to turn his will and his life over to the care of God, and realized that he wanted to live a life based on spiritual principles. He was committed to this new way of life, and to continuing down the path he had chosen. He found that he had to become entirely ready to have God remove all these defects of character. The decision to do so left him feeling empowered; he felt he clearly was on the right path. Being ready did not result in any change in his behavior, however. He had to ask for help. He began the Seventh Step with full recognition that he could not do this himself. Humility had been developing throughout his involvement in this program. He was entirely ready, and he believed that a Power outside of himself existed and would help him, so he got down on his knees repeatedly and asked for the ability to be honest. Nothing happened. He continued to make his request and to address other "shortcomings" as well. He began to live each day with an intention to do God's will to the best of his ability. His life improved and at the same time he began to apologize to people whenever he lied. He chose to apologize and tell the truth, rather than live with another lie. This was very difficult to do, and most people did not understand what he was up to when he revealed the truth, contradicting the fabrication he had previously offered. He found in the beginning that he could only recognize the lie long after the statements were made, but he advanced to a point of sometimes being able to catch himself at mid-sentence and salvage the truth. Over a period of months he developed to the point that he was no longer lying. Then he realized that the dishonest thoughts were no longer the first to come to mind. He felt he was actually getting honest. He made arrangements to talk to a friend who had many more years of sobriety, in order to share the new experience of having honest thoughts. He found, however, that he still hesitated before speaking, just as he used to do in order to assess the situation and give himself enough time to develop a presentable lie. The wise friend pointed out that he had developed beyond the dishonesty that he was so focused on months ago, and that it had been removed. It was now time to start trusting himself due to the gift of relief from habitual dishonesty.

This example reveals one person's progression through these Steps. Participants in Twelve Step programs develop faith and humility as they work the Steps. When they realize the ongoing problems presented by some of their old behaviors and the importance of leading their lives based on spiritual principles, they are faced with the possibility of positive change. Yet they have to give up the controls and surrender to a Higher Power with the belief that that Power will effect these changes. This requires effort. In the example given above, the man had to identify the problem, learn about the solution, prepare himself, ask for help, and then work to change his behavior by forcing himself to apologize and tell the truth whenever he lied. As he accomplished these tasks he also continued to grow and make spiritual development a focus of his daily life. It is in this discipline, living each day with the intention of spiritual growth, that the individual begins to experience change.

The professional can play an important role in helping the individual develop a daily program based on spiritual discipline from which the appropriate attention to these two Steps can naturally extend. These Steps provide the professional with the opportunity to examine humility as well, for it is extremely difficult to address this topic without a personal understanding of the concept. Can clinicians teach someone the importance of humility if they maintain a hierarchical stance, with the professional as "expert in the art of living" and the client somehow lacking? Do the implications of these Steps fit at all with a perspective that suggests that one individual has the answers for the other? This stance provides the client with the unfortunate message that they consistently give themselves while coming out of addiction, that they are "less than." It also suggests that humility may be good for the client, but not the professional. If clinicians can incorporate the principles of these Steps into their therapeutic endeavors, they can enlist people through direct efforts and through modeling this way of life. The individual on a spiritual path may need direction and help in self-examination, but he or she tends to gain much more when the professional recognizes that the belief and surrender associated with these Steps is inherent to any attempts at life change based on spiritual discipline. This is not specific to addiction; these Steps are about human beings attempting to change and grow, with a belief that they and others are in this together: flawed, imperfect, yet able to reach out for help from a Power greater than themselves.

The beauty of these Steps is found in the benefit gained by the individuals who examine themselves, recognize both attributes and liabilities, and then go to the next level to extend themselves in an attempt to develop spiritual discipline. Professionals can be useful in this process of change by helping individuals to accurately examine themselves and honestly identify character defects and life goals. This path is very difficult and encouragement to maintain a new spiritual stance is often needed. The professional is in a powerful position to provide this support, and in so doing, establishes recognition of the importance of the task at hand. The professional can also provide an appropriate understanding of responsibility related to change that can easily be confused as people work these Steps. The individual must take action at the same time they ask for help and use a process of surrender. Often people need to have guidance in regard to the action they must take versus surrender to a Higher Power. Perfectionism is a real trap that many people fall into when they begin this process, and the professional can help in defining appropriate boundaries for change as well as in developing reasonable goals. Expectations can be high, while change is slow, so the professional can also help the person with patience while emphasizing the need for daily discipline. In addition, the professional can be of great help to the client in avoiding some of the other pitfalls inherent to this Step, such as denial of certain problems, blindness to character defects, and attempts to specifically avoid dealing with particular issues. The professional can also have a role in keeping the individual focused on his or her Higher Power, rather than just the individual's own role in the process. To guide someone through these Steps requires that the professional take a stand in regard to the use of a Higher Power to direct life change. Without this understanding the professional can inadvertently work against the very principles of these Steps by attempting to direct behavioral changes based solely on the client's willpower.

The Sixth and Seventh Steps are about dedication to a new set of spiritual beliefs that can result in remarkable life change. The process of change requires recognition, preparation, and a request made to a Higher Power. It is an act of surrender, the results of which are out of the individual's control; his or her own role in the process is limited. The Seventh Step prayer reveals the appropriate emphasis with this statement: "I pray that you now remove from me every single defect of character which stands in the way of my usefulness to you and my fellows."[11] The prayer does not request removal of every single defect of character, nor does it specify those defects or shortcomings that would satisfy the individual, but allows for changes deemed necessary by one's Higher Power. That the outcome is not up to the individual is essential to the surrender associated with these Steps. This is confounding to many participants as well as to therapists, yet it fits with the experience of those who have chosen to "turn their lives over," and to live each day looking for guidance based on spiritual principles. It is another lesson in humility, which is necessary to follow this spiritual path.

> Dear Lord. Untie my hands and deliver my heart from sloth. Set me free from the laziness that goes about disguised as activity when activity is not required of me; and from the cowardice that does what is not demanded in order to escape sacrifice.
>
> Thomas Merton

REFERENCES

1. *Narcotics Anonymous, 5th Ed.* (Van Nuys, CA: N.A. World Services, Inc., 1988) p. 34.
2. *Narcotics Anonymous, 5th Ed.* (Van Nuys, CA: N.A. World Services, Inc., 1988) p. 33.
3. *The Twelve Steps and Twelve Traditions* (New York: Alcoholics Anonymous World Services, Inc., 1988) p.66.

4. *Alcoholics Anonymous, 3rd Ed.* (New York: A.A. World Services, Inc., 1976) pp. 75–76.
5. Bill Pittman and Todd Weber, *Drop the Rock: Removing Character Defects* (Center City, MN: Hazleden, 1993).
6. *The Twelve Steps and Twelve Traditions* (New York: Alcoholics Anonymous World Services, Inc., 1988) p. 68.
7. *The Twelve Steps and Twelve Traditions* (New York: Alcoholics Anonymous World Services, Inc., 1988) p. 67.
8. *Alcoholics Anonymous, 3rd Ed.* (New York: Alcoholics Anonymous World Services, Inc., 1988) p. 60.
9. *The Twelve Steps and Twelve Traditions* (New York: A.A. World Services, Inc., 1976) p. 66.
10. *The Twelve Steps and Twelve Traditions* (New York: Alcoholics Anonymous World Services, Inc., 1988) p. 70.
11. *Alcoholics Anonymous, 3rd Ed.* (New York: A.A. World Services, Inc., 1976) p. 76.
12. *The Twelve Steps and Twelve Traditions* (New York: Alcoholics Anonymous World Services, Inc., 1988) p. 71.
13. *The Twelve Steps and Twelve Traditions* (New York: Alcoholics Anonymous World Services, Inc., 1988) p. 73.
14. Pittman and Weber *Drop the Rock: Removing Character Defects* (Center City, MN: Hazelden, 1993) p. 63.
15. *The Twelve Steps and Twelve Traditions* (New York: Alcoholics Anonymous World Services, Inc., 1988) p. 76.
16. *The Twelve Steps and Twelve Traditions* (New York: Alcoholics Anonymous World Services, Inc., 1988) p. 72.
17. *The Twelve Steps and Twelve Traditions* (New York: Alcoholics Anonymous World Services, Inc., 1988) p. 78.

10

Chapter Ten

Steps Eight and Nine

"Made a list of all persons we had harmed, and became willing to make amends to them all."
"Made direct amends to such people wherever possible, except when to do so would injure them or others."

Up to this point the Steps have focused on the individual: establishing a personal recovery program, and attending to character defects. These two Steps focus on healing relationships, changing the perspective from self to others. This is described as a "selfish program," and in fact the first Seven Steps focus on self in relation to Higher Power. Once a good recovery program has been established with daily spiritual discipline, the individual must begin to look outside the self and examine his or her role in relationships. These Steps provide the opportunity to heal past relationships, allowing the individual to come to a better understanding of all relationships and providing the basis for an improved ability to interact with others. Three tasks are involved: documentation (making another list); becoming willing; and making direct amends. "First, we take a look backward and try to discover where we have been at fault; next we make a vigorous attempt to repair the damage we have done; and third, having thus cleaned away the debris of the past, we consider how, with our new-found knowledge of ourselves, we may develop the best possible relations with every human being we know."[1]

These are the amends Steps, also called the restitution Steps. Amends are much more than an apology, they are considered an opportunity to rectify, correct, and make up for a past wrong. Many people stop the addictive behavior and immediately make apologies, which they have usually done repeatedly during their active addiction, so the apologies lack credibility and are relatively useless. An amends goes well beyond the apology. It reveals the sincere desire to make up for the past, and often includes an act that corrects the past problem in the relationship. For many people, leading a different life based on spiritual principles without the addictive behavior can be an amends in and of itself. Other amends will involve directly paying back material or financial debts, while some require creative solutions such as volunteering time to make up for past offenses.

Making amends presents the opportunity to release the baggage of the past as it pertains to relationships, which provides the individual with another tool to release shame and guilt. This is a recurring theme in the Twelve Steps due to the heavy toll extracted by shame and guilt. Relationships are directly affected by the behaviors of the individual in active addiction such as lying, neglect, theft, or even physical harm. The individual who perpetrates these acts often carries the shame and guilt, eliminating any chance of pursuing an ongoing relationship. The addict will often avoid people they have harmed, unable to face the truth about their past behavior and thus unable to begin a healing process. Several of the Twelve Steps are intended to allow the individual to rid him or herself of shame, guilt and fear by taking responsibility for his or her past actions. These two Steps are an essential component of this process, as they directly address the healing and understanding of relationships. "Our purpose is to achieve freedom from the guilt that we have carried."[2] Freedom from guilt and shame does not come without a great deal of hard work and effort, however. These two Steps ultimately result in directly facing the people one has harmed or maligned, a very difficult task, but one that pays huge dividends for the person willing to take such a risk. These Steps provide the opportunity to establish a framework for healthy relationships. "Learning how to live in the greatest peace, partnership, and brotherhood with all men and women, of whatever description, is a moving and fascinating adventure."[1]

Step 8: "Made a list of all persons we had harmed, and became willing to make amends to them all." ....

Step Eight is part action and part attitude. People are expected to make a list, then become willing. The Step requires making another list, one which will inevitably reiterate some of what was written in the Fourth Step, but many recovering addicts can easily recite a partial list of the persons they harmed with little thought because they carry it with them daily. The memories of harm to others do not easily leave one's consciousness. Thus many people need these Steps to begin a healing process and relieve themselves of the pain related to past events. "We've always had this list inside us; it was burned into our brains. That was the problem."[4] Many people will readily admit that part of their active addiction was related to attempts to repress the painful reality of their past interactions with others. The list is another expression of honest self-examination. To do a complete list is very difficult, and requires a thorough review of relationships and the harm one has caused. "The Eighth Step is not easy; it demands a new kind of honesty about our relationships with other people."[2] This can be a difficult, painful task, as it opens up the old wounds for further evaluation. Some people wonder why they have to do this again, believing they have completed their review with the Fourth and Fifth Steps. They need assurance of the necessity of this task to get outside of themselves and begin to address relationships. These Steps also threaten the self-centered nature of addicts/alcoholics. They must actually look at their own role in relationships. They cannot just focus on themselves, nor can they continue to blame others, if they correctly perform the two expectations of this Step.

This Step continues to emphasize movement in the direction of perfection as one is expected to address "all" of the problems pertaining to relationships. This eliminates the possibility of leaving a few very painful or embarrassing episodes off of the list, forcing the individual to thoroughly examine their past and work toward the ideal willingness necessary to complete the Step. Willingness is an essential aspect of several of the Twelve Steps, but none of the others require it so explicitly as Step Eight. A Twelve Step acronym "HOW" stands for honesty, open-mindedness, and willingness. This saying is used to describe the attitude necessary to work this program, and is specific to Step Eight. To become "willing to make amends to them all" is a difficult task, fraught with fear, because the individual usually has Step Nine in mind and begins to consider facing the individuals to make direct amends. It is important to withhold such thoughts for Step Nine; slow down and make a list, then work toward willingness. Most people view this level of willingness as another form of surrender. One has to accept that the degree of difficulty and pain inherent to this task will be worthwhile in the end. The sharing done by others about the positive results of this Step provides the proof needed to persuade people to willingly forge ahead.

"We might next ask ourselves what we mean when we say we have 'harmed' other people. What kinds of 'harm' do people do one another, anyway? To define the word 'harm' in a practical way, we might call it the result of instincts in collision, which cause physical, mental, emotional or spiritual damage to people."[4] This discussion by Bill Wilson goes on to list several examples of such harm, starting with easily identifiable acts such as lying to and cheating others. He also includes selfish sexual conduct and such acts as paying much more attention to one family member than to another. This is a good description, but once again individual members are left to decide for themselves what harmful acts should make the list. For a problem to register enough concern to enter one's consciousness and make the list requires a thorough, honest review of one's relationships. The identification of "harm" done starts with those acts one carries consciously, the ones that produce consistent worry, shame, or fear. Review of major relationships, including family, friends, and romances will produce acts that may be less obvious, but are just as important. Using the Fourth Step inventory and knowledge from the Sixth Step will provide more examples that need to be added to the list. Most members also discuss the necessity of including oneself on the list of those harmed. The Step suggests that one acknowledges "all" harm caused, ambiguous as it may sound; the member who sincerely and honestly examines interactions with others will be able to come up with a reasonable way of determining what he or she believes to be "harm." A sponsor or a clinician can be of great help to those who find this to be a vague, difficult task, or those who get stuck trying to do too much in a compulsive manner. It is necessary to be thorough and remain open-minded to any possibility of "harm" done others.

There are three main obstacles to this Step: the fear related to directly making amends associated with the Ninth Step, resentment directed toward others, and the inability to witness the harm one has caused. This Step must be considered independent of the Ninth Step in order to make a complete list, and become "willing to make amends to them all." The Eighth Step requires the freedom to develop willingness separate from Step Nine, to avoid being limited by the fear specific to the "direct amends." Without this fear, one can complete the list, and focus on the establishment of willingness, rather than getting caught up in the details of the amends themselves. This also prevents development of "acceptable" versus "unacceptable" amends to make, as this Step is about willingness, not discernment. This is a process, one requiring tremendous willingness before the individual can act upon the amends. Resentment related to past interactions with others can keep the individual from witnessing his or her own role in past difficulties. "To escape looking at the wrongs we have done another, we resentfully focus on the wrongs he has done us."[5] An old saying used in Twelve Step programs suggests that the individual "cleans off their own side of the street." This maintains the focus on self, examining one's own role in the events considered harmful to others, allowing the individual to be accountable for his or her own behavior rather than focusing on someone else. Having completed the prior Steps one would think that denial would no longer be much of an issue, and often this is the case, but admitting one's own problems is remarkably different than examining one's relationships, so elements of denial can continue to veil the truth. "Some of us, though, tripped over a very different snag. We clung

to the claim that when drinking we never hurt anybody but ourselves."[6] Just as Step Four recommended, one must be "searching and fearless" in attempting to discover the harm that has
been caused rather than attempting to justify the behavior.
Professionals well versed in these Steps can direct people to
address and avoid these significant obstacles.

Step Eight provides another opportunity for the individual to
learn about him or herself. The goal is to fully examine relationships, but in a manner specific to the healing of the past. Before a
new way of interacting with others can be established, one must
learn from and heal those issues that continue to plague relationships. This Step allows the member to admit wrongdoing, examine
their role, learn from the past mistakes, and heal the shame and
guilt that also limits their current relationships. "While the purpose
of making restitution to others is paramount, it is equally necessary that we extricate from an examination of our personal
relations every bit of information about ourselves and our fundamental difficulties that we can."[7] Having made a complete list,
the member is in a position to fully examine all manner of defects
specific to relationships. Patterns of behavior and character traits
that interrupt appropriate interactions can be gleaned from such
self-examination. Members who chose to continue down this difficult path are by now quite serious about personal growth, and this
Step provides both a bounty of information about their relationships and the opportunity for healing, so they do not have to continue to make the same mistakes and can begin to alter their
relationships in a thoughtful, positive manner.

Step Eight also engages the member in the process of forgiveness. In order to examine relationships in a manner that reflects
the willingness associated with this Step, one has to consider forgiveness, both of others and of self. "The Eighth Step starts the
process of forgiveness: We forgive others; possibly we are forgiven; and finally we forgive ourselves and learn how to live in the
world"[2] The individual able to examine his or her own role in events
destructive to relationships can witness the healing power of forgiveness. Rather than holding on to resentments, the member is
instructed to focus on his or her own role in the problem relation-

ship. In most cases this provides the proper perspective for the individual to take account of his or her actions rather than those of the other parties. This alters the member's perspective at a time when he or she has been honestly examining many aspects of his or her life, and is more willing to consider forgiveness. This type of forgiveness is akin to acceptance—of oneself and of others. Acceptance of this type relates to being human, "not-God," and capable of atrocities as well as forgiveness.

As mentioned, addiction is a lonely endeavor. The guilt and shame associated with addictive behavior and its consequences limits one's ability to interact with others. As the problems mount, so do the reasons for avoidance. This Step allows for the process of healing to begin so that members can reinvolve themselves with others, and do so in a manner that relieves them of shame and reflects growth and change. "As a result of this Step, we receive a new freedom and can end isolation."[8] Willingness "to make amends to them all" is the attitude necessary for completion of this Step and sets the stage for Step Nine.

Step Nine: "Made direct amends to such people wherever possible, except when to do so would injure them or others."

This is a Step of action that requires tremendous courage. The member is asked to directly address the people they have harmed and to make restitution. The only decision remaining after the Eighth Step is who to leave out, which is differentiated by the possibility of causing further harm. Many members begin recovery with a mad dash to apologize to as many people as they can. Sometimes this is necessary, but it does not always fulfill the expectations of this Step, which suggests an amend, not an apology. "Good judgment, a careful sense of timing, courage, and prudence—these are the qualities we shall need when we take Step Nine."[9] Step Nine requires patience, thoughtful self-examination, and restraint. It is difficult to admit one's mistakes, but to admit mistakes to others and then make amends is a daunting task for the Twelve Step member. Humility, which is emphasized in the Seventh Step, plays a major role in this adventure of healing relationships.

After completion of Step Eight, further preparation is needed for Step Nine. Focus must be maintained on the goal, which is making amends to others, not excusing behavior, blaming others, proving something, or arguing about these events. It is very easy for the member to lose focus and lapse into old thinking, undermining the very nature of this Step. Nor does the individual need to grovel, however. Having embarked on a spiritual path, the task is to live it, which includes amends and other acts of humility, but does not include self-victimization. One must remain centered, praying about one's decisions, and the task at hand. It is useful to involve one's sponsor and others in this task. Support is needed to carry out this Step correctly, and some of the most difficult amends to make will require gaining strength from others. More than anything else one must focus on the people to which the amends will be made, considering each instance carefully and maintaining willingness to do the "next right thing," in spite of the outcome or one's fear of the process.

Using the list from Step Eight one has to determine to whom one must make amends, as well as when and how. "There are those who ought to be dealt with just as soon as we become reasonably confident that we can maintain our sobriety. There will be those to whom we can only make partial restitution, lest complete disclosures do them or others more harm than good. There will be other cases where action ought to be deferred, and still others in which by the very nature of the situation we shall never be able to make direct personal contact at all."[9] Amends should be made to all persons who have been harmed, everyone on the list, unless it will cause further harm. Some amends are needed immediately, and should be addressed as emergent, because postponement would cause even more harm. In these cases one may have to act before fully realizing the potential of this and prior Steps. Partial restitution is often used to address illegal acts or sexual indiscretions that could result in undesirable consequences to others if fully disclosed. Often it is difficult to discern what to do about some of these. The member must attempt to weigh the pain he or she carry versus the harm to another. Timing of the amends is crucial; thus, delay can be used as a tactic to properly address a situation, but one has to be wary of procrastination. Certain people cannot be addressed directly, whether it is due to the circumstances of the relationship, the harm one could cause them or others by "direct amends," or due to death. Situations that do not lend themselves to "direct amends" can still be attended to with indirect amends. Creativity is needed for such circumstances, such as providing anonymous financial gifts or doing volunteer work to make up for such things as past theft.

This Step is very difficult, and most people can find many reasons to avoid "direct amends," thus the emphasis in the Twelve Step literature is to persevere carefully and err on the side of making the amend, always with the intent to avoid harm. By nature, many members find themselves all too willing to drop people off the list. The clinician can be of help in supporting a courageous stance, emphasizing the necessity of carrying out "direct amends" whenever possible. "Above all, we should try to be absolutely sure that we are not delaying because we are afraid. For the readiness to take the consequences of our past acts, and to take responsibility for the well-being of others at the same time, is the very spirit of step Nine."[10] Members often focus on their own feelings of fear, shame and guilt, which can significantly limit their ability to carry out the amends. They view the problem in terms of facing someone else, but just as pertinent, and perhaps more difficult, is the problem of facing themselves. This Step offers freedom from the demons that are associated with other people, revealing the possibility of healthy relationships.

In Twelve Step meetings, discussions of this Step often focus on the incredible results that can occur when "direct amends" are made. Relationships can be renewed and redefined, old wounds can be healed, and freedom from guilt and shame can provide the basis for developing a new way of being in relationships. On occasion the discussion will include amends that have gone awry, but for the most part the discussion is positive and expectations are set for wonderful experiences. It is important for the participant to recognize that they are "responsible for the effort, but not the outcome." One cannot account for the response of the recipients of the amends. Most people will react out of kindness and forgiveness, especially if they witness the willingness and sincerity of effort associated with proper execution of this Step. This can result in a remarkable experience, and reinforces ongoing efforts to make "direct amends." Unfortunately some people have been badly burned by the behavior of the addict, and do not accept the amends, nor wish to even see the member. Under these circumstances the member has to be accepting of the other's wishes, and may need to consider an alternative course, such as an indirect amend. A negative experience should not alter the member's resolve to complete the task and make all the amends necessary. This Step is not done for the individual who is on the receiving end of an amend, it is done for the member to continue a healing process of growth and development in regard to relationships. Positive results will occur even if the experience with a particular amend is not satisfactory.

One member described his experience with this Step as life changing. He was able to free himself from guilt and shame related to certain people, reconnect with people, and come to a new understanding of what it means to be a friend. His initial amends were with family, for they experienced the brunt of the problems related to his addiction, which could be considered a consistent level of harm as they watched him self-destruct. These amends were initiated while he was in treatment, before he even read the Eighth and Ninth Steps. The attempt was primarily an apology, with little in the way of restitution, but he was sincere, unlike the numerous apologies and promises he had made during active addiction. His counselor told him he had much more to do in this regard, but he did not understand it at the time. He entered a Twelve Step program and involved himself with a sponsor who emphasized working the Steps. As he proceeded he began to recognize the importance of spiritual discipline, and was grateful for the direction the Steps provided in regard to personal growth.

As he completed Steps Four through Seven he was faced with some of the harm he had caused others. He found the list associated with Step Eight to be rather easy in that he had several incidents in mind that he could not forget and lamented on what seemed to be a daily basis. He also used the lists he had developed from the Fourth and Sixth Steps. He was willing to change and willing to do whatever the Steps suggested in order to continue to improve upon his life, so willingness to make "direct amends" was in keeping with his understanding of recovery. He perceived Step Nine as a necessary task, and developed a plan to make amends to the people on his list. He met with each of his parents and siblings individually to make amends. This involved a discussion of his life in recovery, an expression of his love for them, and his appreciation of their role in his life. They all received this with enthusiasm, and were very complementary of his endeavors in recovery. He attempted to contact an old girlfriend who refused to speak with him, so he spoke at meetings about the harm he had caused her and found himself able to talk with women in a remarkably new manner. In fact, he could befriend women without considering sexual involvement, and the regret slowly passed. He was frightened to make an amend to the parents of an old friend, so he postponed it, and spoke with his sponsor. He did not want to admit to an act that they had not attributed to him but that had deeply hurt their entire family. Ultimately, he bolstered his courage and went to them. They were shocked but accepting of the amends he proposed, especially after he described his new way of life and the reason behind his visit. He chose not to directly address some store owners from whom he had stolen; he was the primary breadwinner in his new family, and afraid that such an admission could result in a loss of income and thus having severe consequences for his family. He did choose to avoid such behavior and gave of his time and money to a local charity that provided clothing to the poor. He believed that this was an appropriate amend to the community. He began to experience a new freedom with people, which altered his relationships dramatically. With a solid foundation of spiritual discipline and the attention to healing of relationships provided by these two Steps, he has been able to establish intimate, long-lasting relationships that exceed anything he had experienced prior to recovery.

Clinicians can play a major role in directing the member to a new understanding of relationships. Some of the members have had very poor examples of appropriate relationships, coming out of abusive homes and relationships. They may want better relationships but have no idea what this means. If drug and alcohol use was established in early adolescence and continued through young adulthood, they may have missed important social, interpersonal, and individual developmental milestones, limiting their ability to interact with others. The addictive lifestyle can significantly interfere with relationship development. These two Steps provide a blueprint for healing relationships, and encourage examination of relationships, which may be enough for socially adept members to establish a new way of dealing with people. Others will need a clinician to help them to come to understand some of their past experiences and problems with relationships and to support this attempt at establishing a new way of being with others.

The clinician can also support efforts specific to the two Steps, with an understanding of the expectations these Steps have to address all past harm done in relationships. The list itself may exclude some relationship issues that the clinician is aware of and can present to the member. The clinician may be able to help in determining the people to avoid, which requires a working knowledge of the difficulty of these Steps, as well as the ease at which people can convince themselves to skip direct amends. To become willing is a spiritual act, especially as it pertains to the expectation to consider them "all," another example of seeking a degree of perfection that cannot be obtained. Members may need to be reminded that, "No one among us has been able to maintain anything like perfect adherence to these principles. We are not saints. The point is, that we are willing to grow along spiritual lines. The principles we have set down are guides to progress. We claim spiritual progress rather than spiritual perfection."[11]

Most clinicians, especially in psychotherapy, will address the client's relationships, but seldom will they consider an attempt to directly address all the problems the client has ever had in relationships. It is with an understanding of these factors that the clinician must engage the participant in these Steps. These Steps are powerful tools to address guilt and shame, so a clinician adept in their use can support efforts by the individual to rid him or herself of the pain of past relationships that blocks their progress. These Steps turn the members' attention away from themselves to begin the task of healing relationships; they empower the member to risk "direct amends" in order to experience freedom from the past and develop a new understanding of relationships. Clinicians can play an essential role in this process.

Steps Eight and Nine present members with the opportunity to get outside of themselves and turn the focus to other people in their lives. Having completed the prior Steps which focus on self-healing and establishing a spiritual perspective, it is a natural transition to begin to look at relationships. This begins with a review of the past, and a list specific to the "harm" caused others. Once this is accomplished the member is asked to become "willing to make amends to them all." It is in this willingness that the healing process begins. Imagine being willing to make amends for all the harm you have ever produced. It is another example of the accountability emphasized by Twelve Step programs, a statement of intent to clean up all the problems one has ever caused others. Having established this incredible degree of willingness the member is advised to "make direct amends" to the people on the list. This requires courage and resolve, but results in tremendous healing and growth. The member actually attempts to make restitution for the past mistakes. This act relieves the member of tremendous guilt and shame while he or she is learning about appropriate interactions with others, resulting in the ability to establish healthy relationships. The healing of the past allows one to move forward with a new-found freedom in regard to interactions with others, and provides for an end to the isolation of addiction.

REFERENCES

1. *The Twelve Steps and Twelve Traditions* (New York: Alcoholics Anonymous World Services, Inc., 1988) p. 79.

2. *Narcotics Anonymous, 5th Ed.* (Van Nuys, CA: N.A. World Services, Inc., 1988) p. 35.

3. *Sexaholics Anonymous* (Nashville: Sexaholics Anonymous, 1989) p. 123.

4. *The Twelve Steps and Twelve Traditions* (New York: Alcoholics Anonymous World Services, Inc., 1988) pp. 82–83.

5. *The Twelve Steps and Twelve Traditions* (New York: Alcoholics Anonymous World Services, Inc., 1988) p. 80.

6. *The Twelve Steps and Twelve Traditions* (New York: Alcoholics Anonymous World Services, Inc., 1988) p. 81.

7. *The Twelve Steps and Twelve Traditions* (New York: Alcoholics Anonymous World Services, Inc., 1988) p. 82.

8. *Narcotics Anonymous, 5th Ed.* (Van Nuys, CA: N.A. World Services, Inc.,1988) p. 37.

9. *The Twelve Steps and Twelve Traditions* (New York: Alcoholics Anonymous World Services, Inc., 1988) p. 85.

10. *The Twelve Steps and Twelve Traditions* (New York: Alcoholics Anonymous World Services, Inc., 1988) p. 89.

11. *Alcoholics Anonymous, 3rd Ed.* (New York: A.A. World Services, Inc., 1976) p. 60.

Chapter Eleven

Step Ten

"Continued to take personal inventory and when we were wrong promptly admitted it."

Step Ten is the beginning of the maintenance Steps. One through Nine provide a firm foundation for the member who commits to recovery by developing a spiritual program, cleaning up the past, and addressing major defects and relationships. Step Ten is a profound attempt on the part of the member to continually monitor thoughts, words, and behaviors, then "promptly" act on any transgressions. It is much more than an active, ongoing, inventory. This Step is a spiritual discipline, requiring vigilant self-examination, intended to train the member to continually move toward self-improvement. "Every day is a day when we must carry the vision of God's will into all of our activities. 'How can I best serve Thee—Thy will (not mine) be done.' These are thoughts that will go with us constantly."[1] The identification and elimination of current problems is essential to the member seeking a new way of life. In the *Alcoholics Anonymous* text, The Promises directly precede the initial discussion of Step Ten (see pages 41–42). This suggests that a remarkable transformation has taken place as a result of the hard work and discipline associated with the first Nine Steps. The Tenth Step provides the basis for maintaining these gains and is the catalyst for sustained spiritual growth. "We have entered the world of the Spirit. Our next function is to grow in understanding and effectiveness."[2]

This step combines self-examination, in the form of a "personal inventory," with direct amends. It is as if the individual is asked to work the first Nine Steps in real time, pertaining to current activities, in order to experience consistent self-improvement. The addictive diseases are characterized by denial and self-deception. This Step guards against persistent defects or new problems by using a continuous inventory. "The emphasis on inventory is heavy only because a great many of us have never really acquired the habit of accurate self-appraisal."[3] Recognition of defects is a consistent enigma, requiring honest self-examination. The member who has completed the prior Steps should be proficient, and readily able to incorporate such an inventory into their daily discipline.

"A continuous look at our assets and liabilities, and a real desire to learn and grow by this means, are necessities for us."[4] It is recommended that members review their thoughts, words and deeds on a regular basis. The exact form in which this is accomplished is not well defined. Members can use a list of questions to evaluate personal behavior or they can review daily activities to examine their roles and attitudes. An inventory checklist is very helpful in gaining a sense of positive and negative changes that take place over a period of time (see Figure 11-1). A written inventory can offer the additional benefit of an objective record. Some members use a personal journal to complete their inventory. It is essential to evaluate both assets and liabilities to furnish the member with a proper inventory that reveals positive changes and reinforces sustained effort. Timing is a distinguishing factor in regard to the inventory. A "spot check" is used whenever it is needed. If a problem arises during the day, one may use such a method to examine the issue immediately, and respond accordingly. This is often employed to "help in quieting stormy emotions."[5] A daily inventory is suggested in Twelve Step literature, and is the most common technique used. "When we retire at night we constructively review our day."[6] "When evening comes, perhaps just before going to sleep, many of us draw up a balance sheet for the day."[7] Attending to an inventory at the end of each day allows for immediate review of the day's events, provides a system for putting the day behind to eliminate worry, and is consistent with daily spiritual discipline. On occasion, a discussion with one's sponsor

Watch for — X

Month

Year

Check Results DAILY in Proper Column

ASSETS

Strive for — ✔

	1	2	3	4	5	6	7	8	9	10	11	12	13	14	15	16	17	18	19	20	21	22	23	24	25	26	27	28	29	30	31	
Self-Pity																																Self-Forgetfulness
Self-Justification																																Humility
Self-Importance																																Modesty
Self-Condemnation																																Self-Valuation
Dishonesty																																Honesty
Impatience																																Patience
Hate																																LOVE
Resentment																																Forgiveness
False Pride																																Simplicity
Jealousy																																Trust
Envy																																Generosity
Laziness																																Activity
Procrastination																																Promptness
Insincerity																																Straightforwardness
Negative Thinking																																Positive Thinking
Vulgar, Immoral, Trashy Thinking																																High-Minded, Spiritual, CLEAN Thinking
Criticizing																																Look for the GOOD

CHECK THE SCORE EVERY NIGHT

Eliminate the Negative

Made a searching and fearless, moral inventory of ourselves.

Admitted to God, to ourselves and to another human being the exact nature of our wrongs.

Accentuate the Positive

Were entirely ready to have God remove all these defects of character.

Humbly asked Him to remove our shortcomings.

Continued to take personal inventory and when we were wrong, promptly admitted it.

Distributed by *Publishing and Distributing Department*

HAZELDEN / CENTER CITY, MINNESOTA 55012 • (612) 257-7184

Figure 11-1. "My Daily Inventory."

STM 1

or spiritual advisor is an opportunity to do a review of major issues, check on progress, and gain an objective opinion. These can be spontaneous discussions, or done at regular intervals. Some members do an annual inventory to evaluate gains made and to express liabilities in an organized fashion. Twelve Step retreats or renewal centers offer the opportunity to focus on recovery and complete a more involved inventory. These experiences can enhance a person's Twelve Step program, renew commitment, and often provide a sanctuary for intimate sharing. "Having so considered our day, not omitting to take due note of things well done, having searched our hearts with neither fear nor favor, we can truly thank God for the blessings we have received and sleep in good conscience."[8]

This Step also recommends a prompt admission when mistakes are made. This is a continuing effort at restitution consistent with the Eighth and Ninth Steps. It is always difficult to admit one's wrongdoings, but promptly doing so prevents the proliferation of negative emotion that undermines spontaneous human interaction. Prompt attention also reduces the impact on others, enhancing relationships because people recognize an honest, sincere approach to problem solving. In addition to limiting problems, the simple act of apologizing or admitting to wrongdoing becomes remarkably healing. By dealing with these wrongs as they occur, they lose their power, and no longer require energy or attention.

The Tenth Step inventory provides the member with the information needed to identify problems and pursue self-improvement. The daily use of this inventory provides continuous information about the member; it is this recognition that in turn allows the member to specifically direct efforts at growth and change. "Learning daily to spot, admit, and correct these flaws is the essence of character-building and good living. An honest regret for harms done, a genuine gratitude for blessings received, and a willingness to try for better things tomorrow will be the permanent assets we shall seek."[9] For people who are not adept at self-examination, the regular use of an inventory may be the only manner in which they can recognize, address, and learn from the problems that are bound to surface in everyday life. This disciplined effort can result in continuous self-improvement. Another feature of the inventory is the recognition of the rewards of growth and change. The inventory provides a built-in mechanism for evaluating progress. Evidence of growth reinforces the self-enhancing efforts of the member.

As members develop, the problems they face can become dramatically different than those they addressed in early recovery. For most, the problems are of a more subtle nature. I am reminded of a biker who was wrestling with illegal activities for financial gain when he entered a Twelve Step program. A couple of years later he was not engaged in such activities, but found himself concerned about the quality of his relationship with his wife. Peeling the onion skin is frequently discussed in Twelve Step meetings to describe the notion of change as process. One deals with a set of issues, only to find another set of issues to deal with. Fortunately for the member working a rigorous program there is a significant qualitative difference in the level of difficulty and the type of problems being faced; this is one of the miracles of the program. Since the internal emotional response to any level of problem may feel equivalent, an objective examination is necessary to recognize actual growth and development. A regular inventory can provide the member with the objectivity to recognize such differences, as well as the associated advances they have made. This is not always adequate, so the help of a friend, sponsor or clinician may be necessary to point out to the member the exact nature of their progress. Spiritual growth does not completely eliminate human difficulties, but most members working a rigorous program find that their difficulties, and their responses to them, change dramatically over time.

This Step provides the member with a tool to keep his or her side of the street clean. By promptly reacting to wrongs, interpersonal problems are directly addressed and consequences are minimized. A prompt reaction prevents the problem from growing and interfering with relationships. Sometimes the member can identify and respond to a problem immediately by using a spot check inventory, or they identify it later during a daily inventory, which provides the opportunity to take care of it within twenty-four hours. This is the ideal, but it is very difficult to admit to mistakes, so identification is only the beginning of the process. The member must make a courageous decision to face someone directly and admit to a mistake, make an amend, or offer an apology. It is a risk that becomes easier as the member repeatedly experiences positive results. This process enhances relationships, because everyday difficulties are not allowed to fester and interfere. This Step also provides a mechanism of monitoring activities in such a way as to direct attention to improvement of relationships. It is not just about identifying and addressing wrongs; an inventory is also used for self-enhancement. Thus, the member is able to direct efforts to enrich their interactions with others. "Courtesy, kindness, justice, and love are the keynotes by which we may come into harmony with practically anybody."[9]

Sustained improvement is necessary to recovery for Twelve Step members. It is generally accepted that if one is not growing, one is moving backward toward active addiction. This is the motivation for the rigorous spiritual discipline associated with this program. A Tenth Step inventory can identify such gains and losses, thus preventing catastrophe. Emotional and interpersonal problems are considered common reasons for relapse, and thus the member needs to guard against the expansion of such difficulties. The regular use of an inventory is not only for personal growth; it is also a preventive measure. Consistent evaluation and improvement prevents the establishment of patterns of negative behavior that can undermine advances made by working these Steps.

One member described her experience with this Step as essential to her daily life. She uses an inventory every night, even after many years of sobriety. She described the initiation of the Tenth Step after a recommendation by her sponsor when she was struggling with some problems with peers at work. Although she had read the Step, she had never considered an ongoing effort. Once she began, she found it to be immensely helpful in addressing the marked changes she was experiencing. She began with an inventory checklist, which allowed her to review her day using a list of characteristics that she would have had great difficulty determining on her own. She said she needed an outline, something to structure the daily review. Over time this checklist provided visual evidence of those liabilities that continued to be a problem. If she was dishonest for five days in a row, it was there to see every night when she checked dishonesty again. This gave her confidence that she was on the right path, because she could identify problem areas easily, and work to correct them. Attributes were also documented, which supported her self-esteem, and revealed the results of her efforts at self-change. After a period of several months she found she was able to review herself without the checklist, quickly considering most of the same characteristics while she reviewed the major activities of the day. Following the inventory she always prayed for continued help in regard to self-improvement. She also began to act upon the mistakes she made, and when necessary would make a prompt, direct, amend. This left her with fewer liabilities to review, as she took care of many of the potential problems before she got to the inventory. She began to witness tremendous positive changes, and was pleased, but found a few patterns of behaviors that were very stubborn. To address this she started to journal her life experience, both past and present. This provided the ability to examine her daily activities and her emotional reactions in the context of her whole life, while keeping a record that she was able to look back on. She attended an annual retreat for women in recovery and would bring her journal along to review, and then discuss pressing issues in group or individually with her sponsor. In addition to developing skills to recognize and address problems, she found that this Step induced an ability to self-correct and to gain direction for further growth in recovery.

Working with members of Twelve Step programs at this level can be a privilege. They are extremely proactive and fully engaged in personal growth, especially if they are working on this Step. The clinician versed in cognitive behavioral therapy will appreciate certain aspects of this Step. It uses analysis of one's behavior and thought patterns to initiate change. The interventions are thought out and directed toward positive responses. The individual uses a method of self-monitoring on a regular basis, and promptly acts to correct mistakes. The Step can be a useful tool for the clinician in examining life change and growth. If someone is stuck, and cannot determine a strategy to address certain characteristics or behaviors, this Step can be instituted with confidence. It is a fairly simple Step, but attending to a daily inventory is a strict discipline which may need reinforcing, and to perpetually consider self-change and growth can be a bit overwhelming for certain members. The members who have rigorously developed a personal recovery program readily endorse a spiritual approach, emphasizing movement in the direction of perfection while recognizing one's humanity. It is essential for the clinician to recognize this, support the process, and incorporate the Step into any attempts at personal growth.

The Tenth Step is the first of the maintenance Steps, and suggests that the individual following this spiritual path should use a continuous inventory and promptly admit to any wrongdoing. Ongoing self-evaluation is at the heart of any spiritual discipline. The inventory promotes recognition of daily difficulties that can undermine personal growth and provides the impetus for perpetual self-improvement. This is a Step of profound intent, requiring a vigilant, consistent effort. Having completed the first Nine Steps, the member has experienced some remarkable changes. In order to maintain the results of that effort, and continue to experience personal growth, a commitment to self-evaluation must be made. It is done in real time: a problem occurs, it is addressed, and the member moves on without the burden of shame and guilt associated with unfinished emotional affairs. This Step prevents the establishment of problems and provides direction for positive self-change. "For the wise have always known that no one can make much of his life until self-searching becomes a regular habit, until he is able to admit and accept what he finds, and until he patiently and persistently tries to correct what is wrong." [4]

REFERENCES

1. *Alcoholics Anonymous, 3rd Ed.* (New York: A.A. World Services, Inc., 1976) p. 85.

2. *Alcoholics Anonymous, 3rd Ed.* (New York: A.A. World Services, Inc., 1976) p. 84.

3. *Alcoholics Anonymous, 3rd Ed.* (New York: A.A. World Services, Inc., 1976) pp. 91–92.

4. *The Twelve Steps and Twelve Traditions* (New York: Alcoholics Anonymous World Services, Inc., 1988) p. 90.

5. *The Twelve Steps and Twelve Traditions* (New York: Alcoholics Anonymous World Services, Inc., 1988) p. 93.

6. *Alcoholics Anonymous, 3rd Ed.* (New York: A.A. World Services, Inc., 1976) p. 86.

7. *The Twelve Steps and Twelve Traditions* (New York: Alcoholics Anonymous World Services, Inc., 1988) pp. 95–96.

8. *The Twelve Steps and Twelve Traditions* (New York: Alcoholics Anonymous World Services, Inc., 1988) p. 97.

9. *The Twelve Steps and Twelve Traditions* (New York: Alcoholics Anonymous World Services, Inc., 1988) p. 95.

12

Chapter Twelve

Step Eleven

"Sought through prayer and meditation to improve our conscious contact with God *as we understood Him*, praying only for knowledge of his will for us and the power to carry that out."

Step Eleven is the second of the "maintenance Steps," the Steps which are designed to provide ongoing sobriety through daily incorporation of new habits of behavior, thought, and the practice of spiritual discipline. It is the latter two of these three that are specifically addressed by this Step. While Step Ten provides members with a basic guide to conduct in the outer world which helps them attend to the health of their relationships with others, Step Eleven is a guide to conduct in the inner world and speaks to developing and maintaining a relationship with God, or Higher Power. Both Steps, then, chart a course for the formerly isolated addict toward reconnection with both the corporeal and numinous aspects of his or her existence.

Like Step Ten, Eleven does not prescribe a discrete, one-time task, but rather a behavioral shift that is to be strengthened through a regular spiritual practice; this practice is to extend, presumably, for the rest of the member's life. This shift in behavior—the establishment of daily spiritual practice—leads in turn to a shift of focus for the addict from ends to means, from reward to process. The founders considered this cognitive and behavioral shift a crucial condition to avoiding relapse. "What we really have is a daily reprieve contingent on the maintenance of our spiritual condition."[1] Also contingent is the possibility of continual progress toward emotional and psychological health. "Our spiritual condition is the basis for a successful recovery that offers unlimited growth."[2]

This "spiritual maintenance" works by first dismantling the self-obsession of the addict. "Belief in the power of God, plus enough willingness, honesty and humility to establish and maintain the new order of things, were ... essential ... [This was] simple, but not easy; a price had to be paid. It meant destruction of self-centeredness."[3] *The Twelve Steps and Twelve Traditions* quotes a variation on the Prayer of St. Francis, a rare reference to any established religious order (though unattributed as such in the A.A. text), as a model of "selfforgetting":

> Lord, make me a channel of thy peace—that where there is hatred, I may bring love—that where there is wrong, I may bring the spirit of forgiveness—that where there is discord, I may bring harmony—that where there is error, I may bring truth—that where there is doubt, I may bring faith—that where there is despair, I may bring hope—that where there are shadows, I may bring light—that where there is sadness, I may bring joy. Lord, grant that I may seek to comfort rather than to be comforted—to understand, than to be understood—to love, than to be loved. For it is by self-forgetting that one finds. It is by forgiving that one is forgiven. It is by dying that one awakens to Eternal Life. Amen.[4]

The message to the addict is that, as with sobriety, "eternal verities" such as peace, hope, truth, and forgiveness are attainable only to the extent that they are freely offered to others.

"Simple, but not easy"—the founders understood the character of the addict and realized that shifting his or her focus from the self to a Higher Power was a daunting task. For some, "our egos are so self-centered that we would not accept God's will for us without another struggle and surrender."[5] For many members, when they first came to the program "something deep inside us kept rebelling against the idea of bowing before any God."[6] Overcoming this resistance—developing an authentic humility before one's Higher Power—is critical to the practice of Step Eleven.

A Spiritual, Not Religious Program ....

"Striving after God is as natural as breathing. ... The problem was not God; there was something wrong with *us*. Our wrongs had separated us ... from *union* with our God. As a result, our concept of God was wrong, and we were lost to the true God. He was either an avenging tyrant we were afraid to approach, the great Authority Figure, a Santa Claus, or some other reflection of our distorted attitudes and dysfunctional relationships ... [We created] a god to suit our sickness."[7] Twelve Step societies call their programs spiritual rather than religious; most, in fact, take pains to emphasize the distinction. At stake in this is, among other things, inclusiveness. As shall be discussed in Chapter 14 on the Twelve Traditions, Twelve Step programs are open to anyone who desires to stop his or her compulsive behavior. To align with any one religious tradition is to exclude potential members, people in dire need of what the program has to offer, simply because they hold a particular religious belief. This is unacceptable to Twelve Step societies, which staunchly maintain that their programs are for everyone in need of help with his or her addiction.

Another reason for the refusal to align with any religion or sect is that many addicts have had unpleasant experiences with the perceived judgmentalism of some religious traditions; furthermore, many by their nature vehemently resist the idea of a God-concept that is imposed upon them by others. "The experiences that some people talk about regarding meditation and individual religious beliefs don't always apply to us."[8] Twelve Step programs do not in any way disparage the value of any religion or sect, whether established or emerging. Members are supported in whatever form of spiritual expression they may choose. As mentioned, however, Twelve Step societies strongly encourage members to adopt or develop belief systems and spiritual practice that are right for them. They recognize that many addicts are not likely to believe as they are told, particularly when it comes to precepts of right and wrong. "Enforced morality lacks the power that comes to us when we choose to live a spiritual life."[8] Thus, addicts are encouraged in Step Eleven to discover their own sense of moral behavior through consciously asking God for direction and inspiration.

Step Eleven repeats the critical caveat from Step Three regarding the deity: "God *as we understood Him.*" The *Narcotics Anonymous* text goes so far as to refuse to recommend any particular type of meditation in order to protect this concept, stating that to do so "would be a violation of our traditions and a restriction on the individual's right to have a God of his understanding."[8]

To begin to seek conscious contact with "God as we understood Him" requires, for many addicts, that they first begin to build for themselves a new or revised concept of Higher Power that fits their new lives in recovery. Many in active addiction tried vainly to make deals with a God they only vaguely understood and found nothing but an existential silence in response. "No wonder it never worked for us. And no wonder that what we really wanted was to fill the great void at the center of our being and to have a faith that worked." Step Eleven charts a course for the individual toward a "faith that works." "In the Eleventh Step, our lives take on a deeper meaning."[2]

Prayer

While Twelve Step societies carefully avoid telling members *how* to pray, they are explicit in telling them what to pray *for*—and what not to. "When we first come to the program, we usually ask for a lot of things that seem to be important wants and needs. As we grow spiritually and find a power greater than ourselves, we begin to realize that as long as our spiritual needs are met, our living problems are reduced to a point of comfort. When we forget where our real strength lies, we quickly become subject to the same patterns of thinking and action that got us to the program in the first place. ... Sometimes we prayed for our wants and got trapped once we got them."[9]

When addicts first come to Twelve Step programs, the only prayers with which they are familiar are often of the "foxhole" variety: "God, get me through this" or "God, get me out of here." Step Eleven instructs members to pray rather only for knowledge of their Higher Power's will for them and the capacity to fulfill that. Members are of course encouraged to turn to their Higher Power when they are in crisis, but with a different type of prayer that asks for revelation of God's agenda rather than fulfillment of the member's immediate wish. The program suggests only using prayers that petition the Higher Power for requesting help in clearly understanding what exactly *is* God's will, even to the extent of using the prayer "Thy will, not mine, be done" as a kind of practical mantra in times of distress. "Just saying it over and over will often enable us to clear a channel choked up with anger, fear, frustration, or misunderstanding, and permit us to return to the surest help of all—our search for God's will, not our own, in the moment of stress."[10] Over time, members are told, this practice will deliver results. "Most of us pray when we are hurting. We learn that if we pray regularly we won't be hurting as often, or as intensely."[8]

Focusing strictly on the prayer that "God's will, not mine, be done" is frequently necessary for the addict in order for him or her to gain sufficient clarity to differentiate between an intuitive sense of communication with a Higher Power and "well-intentioned unconscious rationalizations."[11] The programs recognize how foreign the concept of conscious contact with God can be for addicts, especially early on in their sobriety, and acknowledge that to members unpracticed in the arts of prayer and meditation, wishful thinking can distort the reception of divine guidance. Rigid or self-serving prayers can lead to, among other pitfalls, a misguided and self-aggrandizing sense of being God's emissary: that one knows more than others or has superior judgment because of one's contact with God, or a belief that one knows God's will for others better than they know it themselves. Twelve Step societies see that kind of prayer as not only self-serving but ineffective in creating the kind of "conscious contact" Step Eleven talks about. Step Eleven—and all of the Steps—are about developing only a *personal* program of recovery. Members are strongly discouraged from (in reference to Step Four) "taking another person's inventory." Thus, when Step Eleven says to pray only for "knowledge of God's will for us," it means only for the individual's knowledge for him or herself. To ask for anything more flirts with exhibiting a desire for power or authority over others; it implies making demands upon God to elevate the individual above others. This, members are told, just does not work. "We discover that we do receive guidance for our lives to just about the extent that we stop making demands upon God to give it to us on order and on our own terms."[12]

Twelve Step programs believe that the practice of prayer over time—for freedom from self-will and to remove internal distractions and blockages that hinder contact with the Higher Power—results in an increasingly sensitive intuitive faculty that is a source of inner strength and emotional sustenance. This in turn allows for even greater willingness to turn one's will and life over to the care of God (Step Three) as trust in the Higher Power expands. Yet even while Step Eleven charts a rigorous and idealistic spiritual regimen for members, the program acknowledges that no one will have anything like perfect compliance, and there will be rough spots along the way. "All of us, without exception, pass through times when we can pray only with the greatest exertion of will. Occasionally we go even further than this. We are seized with a rebellion so sickening that we simply won't pray. When these things happen we should not think too ill of ourselves. We should simply resume prayer as soon as we can, doing what we know to be good for us."[13]

Meditation

Meditation is often a foreign and uncomfortable prospect for addicts. For many, the concept of going within and quieting the mind for a period of time is beyond not only the scope of their experience but of their imagination as well. The *Sexaholics Anonymous* text calls them "noisy souls." The rush of thoughts and images that clatter in their consciousness throughout each day seems normal to them and life without it strange and even frightening. "Most of us coming into [the program] seem to have our inner being filled with noise much of the time. Pollution. We may not be aware of this at first since it built up gradually over the years and we don't sense it as abnormal. ... Being what we are— addicts—this has become a part of our illness. It seems unnatural to be without it." This inner noise is not random—it has a purpose. "This noise helps distract us from our own spiritual discord—a noise all its own—and also feeds this discord."[14]

Meditation is the practice of learning to break through the noise and distraction, to calm the wild rush of thoughts and sensations that mask true feelings and block the simple awareness that one even *has* an inner life, and to then slowly replace it with an inner harmony far more subtle and profound than anything the addict has ever experienced. One of the first benefits is a taming of the emotions. "Emotional balance is one of the first results of meditation."[5] But this process takes time and diligence on the part of the member, and patience and persistence are required. As patience and persistence are not always the addict's strong suits—one humorous prayer addicts wryly offer is "God grant me patience, but grant it to me *now*"— the clinician can do the Twelve Step member a great service by assisting him or her in reinforcing these qualities through treatment goals. Chances are good that members will receive understanding support in this area in their meetings from others who have experienced similar struggles. "We should remind ourselves that skilled people were not born with their skills. It took lots of effort on their part to develop them."[5]

A Practical Spirituality

As esoteric as Step Eleven may sound to those outside Twelve Step societies, members see it as eminently practical. The promised result of practicing Step Eleven is greater peace of mind, greater connectedness with both the seen and the unseen worlds, and nothing less than a sense of belonging in the universe.

Addicts accustomed to the pursuit of immediate gratification will not long persist in an activity that does not produce positive results sooner or later. Most who practice Step Eleven faithfully, however, report greater personal strength, increased energy, a marked decrease in fear and distrust, and a greater acceptance of the world and others. "We become willing to let other people be who they are without having to pass judgment on them. The urgency to take care of things isn't there anymore. We couldn't comprehend acceptance in the beginning; today we can."[15] Over time, those who practice this Step with regularity report that God's will for them slowly begins to merge with their own will for themselves; that is, the intuitive guidance they become increasingly in tune with directs them to think and behave in ways that begin to feel natural. "What used to be a hunch or the occasional inspiration gradually becomes a working part of the mind."[16]

Surrendering one's will to an unseen power and trusting that it will guide one through both mundane daily activities and the inevitable crises that all people encounter to some degree in life—death of loved ones, divorce, business failure, and other key losses and major life changes—requires tremendous faith. Step Eleven asks a great deal of the Twelve Step group member. If the member has rigorously worked the preceding ten Steps, however, he or she is prepared to embark on the adventure of living life along spiritual lines, the life promised by Step Eleven. "God will not force his goodness on us, but we will receive it if we ask."[8] By asking for the help of their Higher Power, however they may define or conceptualize or name it, members are promised—and they expect—that "the answers will come if your own house is in order."[17]

Cognitive–Behavioral–Spiritual

The change in thinking and behavior effected in addicts by sincere practice of the Twelve Steps could be described as cognitive–behavioral–spiritual. The process of change can be charted in five developmental phases, each phase dependent on the one that precedes it.

Phase 1: The first phase is cognitive in nature. The addict makes a conscious choice to accept the very basic spiritual premises of the program: that some spiritual power greater than the addict exists; that it can restore the addict to a state of mental and emotional health; and that the addict has access to the help of this power at all times, provided he or she incorporates a particular, persistent spiritual discipline into his or her life. This is an act of conscious faith in the wisdom of the program and the other addicts and alcoholics for whom the program seems to be working. Sometimes this conscious faith does not meet the criteria to be called belief in the spiritual premises of the program. In such cases, members are encouraged to "act as if" they believed. Belief, they are told, will come later.

Phase 2: This phase is behavioral. Whether acting according to a new, consciously chosen faith or "acting as if," the member begins to put into practice the spiritual regimen prescribed in Step Eleven. He or she starts experimenting with prayer, working to refine the prayers into variations on "Thy will, not mine, be done." As the member continues to work the Step, the practice of prayer becomes increasingly regularized so that the member turns to his or her Higher Power for life guidance at set times of the day as well as when facing a conflict, dilemma, or challenge. The member also begins the practice of meditation, working to develop the mental and emotional skills necessary to quiet the mind and enter a receptive state of consciousness at set times of the day. The rewards of such behaviors are initially quite subtle and may not even be perceived by addicts whose use of psychotropic substances or behavior has accustomed them to sensory gratification both powerful and instantaneous. Their ability to persist in the new practice of spiritual discipline will depend on support from fellow members, clinicians, and in some cases, family, as well as on the extent of their desire for recovery. This is one of the reasons why Twelve Step programs strongly emphasize attendance at meetings: "Keep coming back," newcomers are repeatedly told, "because it works if you work it."

Phase 3: The third phase is a highly personal, subjective experience of a spiritual nature. Practitioners of Step Eleven are told they will begin to develop and refine an intuitive ability that is the "conscious contact with God as we understood Him" promised in the Step. This intuition serves to guide the member through the challenges of day-to-day life.

Phase 4: As the member learns to recognize this intuitive guidance and honor it by following its gentle dictates, the success that results reinforces both the trust in the Higher Power and the wisdom of the Twelve Step approach. Phase four, then, is again cognitive in nature: the member recognizes in a new and deeper way that he or she is connected to the world and to the universe; that there is an unseen power that has his or her best interests at heart and which is available to the member to the extent that it is sought. Furthermore, the member concludes that in such a universe, the member's life must have some meaning and value. Self-esteem is bolstered, the member becomes increasingly peaceful, and sobriety becomes an acceptable and even desirable way of life. Damaged relationships begin to heal, and new, healthy relationships are initiated. The member makes an internal shift in his or her belief system from seeing a universe that is chaotic, dog-eat-dog, random, and uncaring to one that, despite all worldly appearances of conflict, strife, and pain to the contrary, has an underlying order and meaning—a grace—that is both refuge and shepherd.

Phase 5: As members begin to find a new inner peace and outward success in healing relationships through the practice of Step Eleven, the behaviors of recovery—abstinence, rigorous honesty, admitting wrongs promptly, practicing prayer and meditation, attending meetings and continuing to work the Steps, accepting what cannot be changed and changing what can, and carrying the message to others in pain—are reinforced. It is at this stage in recovery that the member feels his or her will is becoming congruent with the will of the Higher Power, and the Promises of recovery found in the Big Book begin to come true:

> If we are painstaking about this phase of our development, we will be amazed before we are half way through. We are going to know a new freedom and a new happiness. We will not regret the past nor wish to shut the door on it. We will comprehend the word serenity and we will know peace. No matter how far down the scale we have gone, we will see how our experience can benefit others. That feeling of uselessness and self-pity will disappear. We will lose interest in selfish things and gain interest in our fellows. Self-seeking will slip away. Our whole attitude and outlook upon life will change. Fear of people and of economic insecurity will leave us. We will intuitively know how to handle situations which used to baffle us. We will suddenly realize God is doing for us what we could not do for ourselves.[18]

REFERENCES

1. *Alcoholics Anonymous, 3rd Ed.* (New York: A.A. World Services, Inc., 1976) p. 85
2. *Narcotics Anonymous, 5th Ed.* (Van Nuys, CA: N.A. World Services, Inc., 1988) p. 41.
3. *Alcoholics Anonymous, 3rd Ed.* (New York: A.A. World Services, Inc., 1976) pp. 13–14.
4. *The Twelve Steps and Twelve Traditions* (New York: Alcoholics Anonymous World Services, Inc., 1988) pp. 101–102.
5. *Narcotics Anonymous, 5th Ed.* (Van Nuys, CA: N.A. World Services, Inc., 1988) p. 43.
6. *The Twelve Steps and Twelve Traditions* (New York: Alcoholics Anonymous World Services, Inc., 1988) p. 99.
7. *Sexaholics Anonymous* (Nashville, TN: Sexaholics Anonymous, 1989) p. 136.
8. *Narcotics Anonymous, 5th Ed.* (Van Nuys, CA: N.A. World Services, Inc., 1988) p. 42.
9. *Narcotics Anonymous, 5th Ed.* (Van Nuys, CA: N.A. World Services, Inc., 1988) pp. 44–45.
10. *The Twelve Steps and Twelve Traditions* (New York: Alcoholics Anonymous World Services, Inc., 1988) p. 104.

11. *The Twelve Steps and Twelve Traditions* (New York: Alcoholics Anonymous World Services, Inc., 1988) p. 106.
12. *The Twelve Steps and Twelve Traditions* (New York: Alcoholics Anonymous World Services, Inc., 1988) p. 107.
13. *The Twelve Steps and Twelve Traditions* (New York: Alcoholics Anonymous World Services, Inc., 1988) p. 108.
14. *Sexaholics Anonymous* (Nashville, TN: Sexaholics Anonymous, 1989) pp. 138–139.
15. *Narcotics Anonymous, 5th Ed.* (Van Nuys, CA: N.A. World Services, Inc., 1988) p. 45.
16. *Alcoholics Anonymous, 3rd Ed.* (New York: A.A. World Services, Inc., 1976) p. 87.
17. *Alcoholics Anonymous, 3rd Ed.*, (New York: A.A. World Services, Inc., 1976) p. 164.
18. *Alcoholics Anonymous, 3rd Ed.* (New York: A.A. World Services, Inc., 1976) pp. 83–84.

13

Chapter Thirteen

Step Twelve

"Having had a spiritual awakening as the result of these steps, we tried to carry this message to alcoholics, and practice these principles in all our affairs."

The Twelfth Step is a statement of the extraordinary outcome of the first eleven Steps as well as a projection of the ongoing responsibility of the members, to themselves and others. It begins with the declaration of a "spiritual awakening" based on completion of the prior Steps, affirming the experience of members who have rigorously followed this path. This is also a maintenance Step, like Ten and Eleven, which promote means of enriching conduct in the external world (relating to others) and in the internal world (connecting with a Higher Power). Step Twelve suggests two tasks essential to the maintenance of one's spiritual condition: "carry this message" and "practice these principles in all our affairs." This is the ultimate action Step: it suggests continuous attention to spiritual growth and development based on these principles. "The joy of living is the theme of A.A.'s Twelfth Step, and action is the key word."[1] This statement opens the chapter on Step Twelve in *Twelve Steps and Twelve Traditions*. The joy appears to emanate from all three aspects of this Step—a spiritual awakening, carrying the message to others, and practicing the principles. For the member who has advanced through the Steps it is no longer about the marked problems they have experienced as a result of their addiction. Their program is now thoroughly ensconced in spiritual growth; and while spiritual growth requires the foundation of abstinence, this is no longer its sole focus. "Staying sober is our initial objective; a spiritual awakening is the unintended result."[2]

"The result of these steps" is a "spiritual awakening." "When a man or a woman has a spiritual awakening, the most important meaning of it is that he has now become able to do, feel, and believe that which he could not do before on his unaided strength and resources alone. He has been granted a gift which amounts to a new state of consciousness and being."[3] When Twelve Step members discuss what they mean by a spiritual awakening they primarily offer their stories, rich with descriptions of the changes that have taken place in their lives. It is an extremely personal experience, usually only recognized in retrospect. In fact, other people may notice the changes before the member is even aware of any. Bill Wilson described a sudden, miraculous, experience, but most members seem to identify more with the description in "Spiritual Experience," Appendix II of *Alcoholics Anonymous*: "Most of our experiences are what the psychologist William James calls the 'educational variety' because they develop slowly over a period of time." A spiritual awakening can be referred to as a gift that manifests as an astonishing alteration of consciousness that provides the individual with a new awareness, faith, and trust in a Higher Power that plays an active role in their daily life. This is a tremendous transformation, affecting one's entire life perspective. It is in the mind of the beholder, but recognizable to those who have witnessed inexplicable joy emanating from a person who had once depicted ultimate despair. Although a "spiritual awakening" is not readily described, it is pronounced "as the result of these steps." The member works the Steps with this outcome in mind, fully aware of the expected transformation from the stories described by peers. They count on such an experience as they rigorously work the first eleven Steps.

Some members tire or lose sight of the process. They look too hard for "the results" and quit actively working the Steps. It is in the working of the Steps that one effects transformation, not in thinking about the Steps, thinking about a Higher Power, or even remaining abstinent. Step Twelve describes "the results" in the past tense—"*having had* a spiritual awakening as the result of these steps" (italics added)—revealing a precise path to this experience. The Steps are suggested, but the results cannot be attained without conscientiously working them. This can be confusing and frustrating to the member who is abstinent, attending meetings, and working some of the Steps, or working the Steps in a deficient manner. In *Twelve Steps and Twelve Traditions*, there is a description of "two stepping," going from Step One to the Step Twelve. Members who do this limit their Twelfth Step to carrying the message. This is relatively common, and ineffective in gaining all that is to be offered from this program. A modern corollary of "two-stepping" could be called "six stepping." Members who have completed the first five Steps in a treatment program, with little ongoing effort, will begin to work with others in an attempt to "carry the message." Working with others is essential to one's own sobriety and should not be restricted, but members who lose sight of the whole program and do not complete all the Steps will often find themselves dismayed that they have not received the entire benefit of the program. Under these circumstances they need someone (a fellow member, sponsor, or clinician) to direct them to complete all the Steps, and then examine the outcome. "The results" require a specific effort, working all the Steps.

"Helping others is the foundation stone of your recovery."[4] The founding moment of A.A., when Bill W. shared his story with Dr. Bob, reveals the roots of this idea (see Chapters 2 and 3). From the beginning, carrying the message was considered essential to sobriety; in fact, it was this concept that brought the founders together. Bill Wilson believed that sharing the message of one's sobriety would keep one sober. "Practical experience shows that nothing will so much insure immunity from drinking as intensive work with other alcoholics."[5] This is at the heart of the Twelfth Step. The intent of Twelfth Step work is to sustain the member who offers the assistance, despite the fact that the focus appears to be on the person in need of help. A common Twelve Step saying summarizes this concept, "You have to give it away to keep it."

A traditional Twelfth Step call involves a member of a group visiting someone who is actively addicted. A Twelfth Step call is based on "one alcoholic talking with another" in a manner that avoids lecturing, advice, even expertise. It is recommended that the sharing consist primarily of one's story: "what it was like, what happened, and what it's like now." Often the call is made on someone who has never actively pursued help and is not necessarily interested in having someone else tell him or her they have a problem. By maintaining a description of one's own experience the member can avoid provoking a defensive stance, and perhaps even provide information that the person recognizes. "You can help when no one else can."[5] It is always emphasized that the member keeps in mind that they are doing this to help themselves. It is all too easy to focus on the suffering addict and lose sight of this. Once again the member is responsible for the effort and not the outcome. It is stated that Twelfth Step work is successful when the member comes away sober. In spite of the emphasis on oneself associated with this part of the Step, there is great joy in helping a fellow alcoholic or addict. "Practically every A.A. member declares that no satisfaction has been deeper and no joy greater than in a Twelfth Step job well done."[6]

There are other types of Twelfth Step work; members can "carry this message" in numerous ways. The member who looks and acts remarkably different than he or she did during active addiction is an example of hope for those who knew him or her in that state, becoming a living example of the benefits of the program. Attending meetings and sharing one's "experience, strength, and hope" is a form of carrying the message that is often overlooked. The newcomer needs to witness the results of the program to be able to commit to it. Members who open the meeting room, make the coffee, set up the chairs, greet others, and clean up are all doing Twelfth Step work. The "trusted servants" who run meetings, administer groups, and volunteer their time at the local, state, and national level are carrying the message. Members who visit hospitals and treatment centers are providing an important service. Twelfth Step work is considered any activity in which the member is performing a service to other addicts, whether they are actively using or clean and sober. The traditional Twelfth Step call and all of these Twelfth Step activities are executed from the heart of one who has been there, and acknowledges the gifts received so freely from other members. "Here we turn outward toward our fellow alcoholics who are still in distress. Here we experience the kind of giving that asks no rewards."[1] Twelfth Step work is compensated with the joy one receives from helping others, and with the reinforcement realized in one's recovery program.

The Twelfth Step states that members "practice these principles in all our affairs." It is the summation of the entire program, recommending use of the Steps in all of one's activities. This statement is consistent with the teachings of the world's great religions and the perennial philosophy in that one is to consider spiritual beliefs as integral to life itself. Bill Wilson uses numerous examples in *Twelve Steps and Twelve Traditions* to demonstrate how alcoholics have dramatically changed by working these Steps in all walks of life and in all their affairs. The initial goal of anyone coming into a Twelve Step program is to stop the pain and the problems related to the addictive behavior. Little do they know that they are beginning a spiritual path that has the potential to alter every aspect of their lives.

The practice of these principles begins in A.A. meetings, where the newcomer witnesses the results of these Steps demonstrated by seasoned members. Those who work the Steps rigorously begin to change and find that they want more, and this "simple program" offers much more. They pursue spiritual growth and develop spiritual disciplines, with the recognition that this program is about their entire life, not just limited to staying sober. The Promises from *Alcoholics Anonymous* reveal some of the qualities one can expect to manifest as a result of working the Steps. The last three Steps develop a maintenance plan for continuous evolution. Of these, the Twelfth explicitly states the ideal, to "practice these principles in all our affairs." A goal stated in spiritual terms, impossible for a human being to attain, yet the perfect model to work toward. This can be of concern to the newcomer, who may need guidance to avoid being overwhelmed. The Steps make several statements of this nature, expressing the ideal for alcoholics who entered the program out of hopelessness and vulnerability. The recognition of limitations provided by Twelve Step programs results in acceptance of one's humanity and that one is "not God." This act of surrender allows members to rely on a Higher Power— and each other—to survive. Thus, the ability to strive for ideal, spiritual objectives is the result of acceptance of limitation, and surrender to a "Power greater than ourselves." It is with this perspective that members accept the implications and challenges of Step Twelve.

Executing this Step in its entirety requires vigilant attention to one's thoughts and behavior. Again, members are asked to strive for perfection, while recognizing human limitation. They cannot escape the implications of this Step, which suggests continuous self-monitoring. Some members discuss the "narrow path" of recovery; they no longer allow themselves the latitude of thought and behavior that they once did. This leaves them consistently striving for self-improvement, which helps to explain the lengths members will go to address their lives. Twelve Step members are seekers and place a high value on personal growth. They incorporate many and varied attempts at self-enhancement. Members frequently use religious involvement to further spiritual development. The inclusive nature of the program helps in limiting problems with various religions. Members attend retreats and conferences. They read self-help books and attend lectures by the authors. They readily involve themselves in psychotherapy to address issues specific to personal growth or coexisting problems. All of these attempts to advance self-understanding and enhance their lives are done in the spirit of Step Twelve.

Ignoring Step Twelve limits the joy of recovery and can quickly contribute to backsliding. "When we first begin to enjoy relief from our addictions, we run the risk of assuming control of our lives again. We forget the agony and pain that we have known. Our disease controlled our lives when we were using. It is ready and waiting to take over again. We quickly forget that all our past efforts at controlling our lives failed."[7] When members do not "practice these principles in all our affairs" they run the risk of going back to what they once were, lacking the recognition of limitation and without spiritual discipline. This can quickly undermine the tremendous advances they have made. They may remain abstinent and yet witness the recurrence of character defects that undermine peace of mind and reintroduce despair. Unfortunately, relapse and the return to the tragedy of addiction becomes a significant risk.

The ultimate goal of the Twelve Steps is to develop and maintain a life based upon spiritual principles. This can drastically alter the course of the member's life and motivates an inquiry into one's deepest held beliefs and value systems. This often results in a reexamination of one's definition of success. Many people do not equate material success with spiritual success, and thus a clash of culturally accepted and spiritually directed goals can occur. "Our desires for emotional security and wealth, for personal prestige and power, for romance and for family satisfactions—all of these have to be tempered and redirected. We have learned that the satisfaction of instincts cannot be the end and aim of our lives. If we place instincts first, we have got the cart before the horse; we shall be pulled backward into disillusionment. But when we are willing to place spiritual growth first—then and only then do we have a real chance."[8] The member devoted to a spiritual path continues to live in the world, and must determine a manner of doing so that is in keeping with his or her new beliefs. "Service, gladly rendered, obligations squarely met, troubles well accepted or solved with God's help, the knowledge that at home or in the world outside we are partners in a common effort, the well-understood fact that in God's sight all human beings are important, the proof that love freely given surely brings a full return, the certainty that we are no longer isolated and alone in self-constructed prisons, the surety that we need no longer be square pegs in round holes but can fit and belong in God's scheme of things—these are the permanent and legitimate satisfactions of right living for which no amount of pomp or circumstance, could possibly be substitutes. True ambition is not what we thought it was. True ambition is the deep desire to live usefully and walk humbly under the grace of God."[9]

Clinicians can readily identify numerous ways in which they can be of benefit to members working the Twelfth Step. The most likely role is in providing guidance and therapy for those seeking assistance in self-understanding and self-improvement. The members need clinicians that comprehend the principles of these Steps and can affirm their struggles with the more difficult aspects of spiritual development. They also may need help understanding how to expand or limit their attempts at self-care, especially faced with the expectation of addressing "all" their affairs. The complexities of examining beliefs and value systems lend themselves to professional assistance. It is beneficial to be able to assess a member's involvement in recovery with a thorough understanding of these Steps. If a member has not adequately completed the prior Steps, it is unlikely they will experience the "spiritual awakening" as promised. The maintenance related to the Twelfth Step—carrying the message and practicing the principles—needs be taken into account when dealing with an unfulfilled member. It should be noted that the commitment to these later Steps must be evaluated, even in those who profess adequate knowledge. Many members do not sufficiently work the Steps, but have great difficulty admitting this. Without reasonable knowledge on the part of the clinician, this will go undetected, and an opportunity to direct the member to participate in a simple, specific solution will be lost.

Satisfactory completion of the prior Steps fulfills the incredible promise of the Twelfth Step, a "spiritual awakening." The Twelfth Step itself suggests two means of maintaining life based on spiritual principles: "carry this message" and "practice these principles in all our affairs." The members of Twelve Step programs gain immensely from helping others; in fact, as mentioned, it is suggested that they cannot keep their own sobriety without giving it away. The later section of this Step advises the member to strive for an ideal, spiritual, objective. This is a profound summary of the Twelve Steps, expressing the route to a joyful, spiritual existence. The Twelfth Step reveals that all the Steps are necessary to experience a "spiritual awakening"; to maintain it the member has to carry the message and perpetually consider these spiritual principles. One needs to become spiritually fit and give it away in order to stay spiritually fit. "Faith without works is dead."[10]

REFERENCES

1. *The Twelve Steps and Twelve Traditions* (New York: Alcoholics Anonymous World Services, Inc., 1988) p. 109.
2. *Sexaholics Anonymous* (Nashville, TN: Sexaholics Anonymous, 1989) p. 143.
3. *The Twelve Steps and Twelve Traditions* (New York: Alcoholics Anonymous World Services, Inc., 1988) p. 110.
4. *Alcoholics Anonymous, 3rd Ed.* (New York: A.A. World Services, Inc., 1976) p. 97.
5. *Alcoholics Anonymous, 3rd Ed.* (New York: A.A. World Services, Inc., 1976) p. 89.
6. *The Twelve Steps and Twelve Traditions* (New York: Alcoholics Anonymous World Services, Inc., 1988) p. 113.
7. *Narcotics Anonymous, 5th Ed.* (Van Nuys, CA: N.A. World Services, Inc., 1988) p. 46.
8. *The Twelve Steps and Twelve Traditions* (New York: Alcoholics Anonymous World Services, Inc., 1988) p. 118.
9. *The Twelve Steps and Twelve Traditions* (New York: Alcoholics Anonymous World Services, Inc., 1988) p. 129.
10. *Alcoholics Anonymous, 3rd Ed.* (New York: A.A. World Services, Inc., 1976) p. 88.

14

Chapter Fourteen

The Twelve Traditions

The Twelve Traditions were first published in the *A.A. Grapevine* as "Twelve Suggested Points for A.A. Tradition" in April 1946. The Traditions resulted as "the fellowship of Alcoholics Anonymous learned to apply its program to itself" throughout the decade of the 1940s.[1] The Twelve Traditions serve as guidelines for both group activity and individual behavior in relation to the group, providing structure for the entire organization in a manner that focuses on carefully limiting the power of both group and individual rather than extending either of them. Just as the Twelve Steps provide the individual with a suggested plan of action directing him or her toward certain ideals of thought and behavior, so do the Twelve Traditions direct the group toward the ideal. They may be considered a spiritual program for the Twelve Step group.

The Twelve Traditions developed out of necessity in response to the rapidly increasing number of meetings starting up throughout the country in the 1940s. As increasing numbers of new groups sought guidance about the fellowship and how it worked, and particularly about practical and procedural concerns pertaining to how the meetings should be run, Bill W. and the New York office found themselves inundated with letters asking for help. As Bill responded to these letters based on his and others' experiences of A.A. meetings, he began to notice a pattern in the types of concerns that arose time and again as well as uniformity to his responses. These emerging ideas were presented in the

Grapevine article. Shortly thereafter, the narrative of the article was condensed to twelve brief statements of principle that paralleled the structure of the Steps. Just as the Twelve Steps taught the alcoholic that he or she was "not-God," and urged reliance on a Higher Power, so too did the Twelve Traditions serve to remind A.A. groups and the home office that they were "not-God" either, and that they, too, had to rely on the direction of a Higher Power as it revealed itself through the "group conscience." In order to protect the organization from itself as well as from the potential destructive grandiosity that characterized many alcoholics—even those in recovery—Wilson and his colleagues codified an organizational philosophy that was in many ways the complete reverse of standard thinking, then and now, on how to design an institution. It has, nonetheless, worked brilliantly to maintain A.A.—and other Twelve Steps groups that have adopted variations on the traditions—as a vital, growing fellowship with a singleness of purpose: to help the suffering alcoholic.

Tradition One: "Our common welfare should come first; personal recovery depends upon A.A. unity."

Tradition One reiterates the fundamental unit of the organization—one alcoholic talking to another—and establishes this idea in a call for unity based on a single-minded attention to the common ground all members share: a desire to stop drinking or using to be effected through mutual aid. This reinforces the central idea that Twelve Step group members are all in the struggle to find sobriety through spiritual growth together. A.A. recognizes in this Tradition the power of the sharing that takes place in the group as all that stands in the way of relapse, rapid deterioration, and premature death for the addict. Thus, it emphasizes the primacy of the unified group as the most essential condition of individuals finding recovery. "The unity of Alcoholics is the most cherished quality our society has."[2] This tradition also serves to balance a structure that, as shall be discussed, favors individual autonomy to an extent that can appear to suggest "sheer anarchy."[3]

Clinicians who recognize the value of Twelve Step group sharing to help the client stay focused on his or her personal growth in sobriety can provide significant support for the client's regular attendance at Twelve Step meetings. The clinician may also remind the client that the dynamic is mutual-help rather than self-help and that committed, on-going participation in Twelve Step meetings serves not only to keep the client in recovery but to help fellow group members do the same.

Tradition Two: "For our group purpose there is only one ultimate authority—a loving God as He may express Himself in our group conscience. Our leaders are but trusted servants; they do not govern."

This tradition clearly expresses the spiritual perspective of the Steps in a group format. While the individual's "power greater than ourselves" can be anything the member chooses it to be—a doorknob, the group, the Twelve Step organization, or an omniscient, beneficent universal intelligence—Tradition Two characterizes the group's higher power more narrowly: "a loving God" expressed in the "group conscience." While this leaves the door open to the atheist or agnostic member to bypass "the loving God" part and just accept the "group conscience" as the only A.A. authority, Tradition Two may represent the most overtly spiritual statement in the Steps and Traditions.

By placing ultimate authority in God as revealed through the group, Tradition Two helps members focus on their personal efforts at developing spiritual discipline and maintaining sobriety by removing all temptation in the form of garnering personal power. No member has power over another member or over the group, not even leaders at the group, intergroup, or national levels. This Tradition turns the standard hierarchical corporate organizational structure upside down by specifically limiting the role of the leaders. "They are servants. Theirs is the sometimes thankless privilege of doing the group's chores."[4] Thus, there is no office to which the member can aspire that places him or her above anyone else in the fellowship—Twelve Step societies have no CEO or president who manages the organization from the top down. Rather, group members rely on the Higher Power to guide them. They expect that a Higher Power will provide answers through the conscience of the group, and they respect the answers received in that manner.

The groups are, then, fundamentally egalitarian, though not necessarily democratic. "There is often a vast difference between group conscience and group opinion, as dictated by powerful personalities or popularity."[5] Tradition Two, as with the Steps, seeks to express the highest ideals for members to try to achieve. For example, early in A.A.'s history, Bill Wilson was offered a professional position as lay therapist at the Charles B. Towns hospital. The hope was that he would transfer his A.A. work there as a for-profit treatment modality, but his A.A. colleagues were skeptical. When Bill assured them it would be completely ethical, another member replied, "Sure, it's ethical, but what we've got won't run on ethics only; it has to be better. . . . This is a matter of life and death [and] . . . sometimes the good is the enemy of the best."[6] Bill turned down the offer, and this is considered one of the earliest examples of the group conscience prevailing as A.A.'s highest authority.

As mentioned, addiction is an isolating disease; conversely, recovery is largely about making connections with others and learning to consider the best interests of others and of the whole. Clearly, Tradition Two supports the therapeutic aims of clinicians trying to help addicted clients. Living up to the ideals of this Tradition requires empathy, patience, sensitivity to the needs of others and the promptings of one's intuition (or conscience), and sublimation of one's own ego needs for the good of the whole.

Tradition Three: "The only requirement for A.A. membership is a desire to stop drinking."

Tradition Three again decentralizes the organizational authority by stating that only the individual can determine whether he or she is qualified to be a member of the Twelve Step program. "You are an A.A. member if you say so. You can declare yourself in; nobody can keep you out. No matter who you are, no matter how low you've gone, no matter how grave your emotional complications—even your crimes—we still can't deny you A.A. . . . You're an A.A. member the minute you declare yourself."[7] This Tradition evolved from negative experiences in the early years of A.A. when some early groups excluded members based on numerous factors and various differences. Some early groups wanted only something called "pure alcoholics" as members. They feared that if some members were not "pure alcoholics," the program would not work for any of them and they would all be doomed to return to active addiction. This point of view was rejected in favor of welcoming all alcoholics based solely on self-diagnosis and their personal motivation—"the desire to stop." "Desire is the key word; desire is the basis of our recovery."[8] Anyone with such a desire is welcome in the Twelve Step fellowship, and all are equal. It is the sole responsibility and choice of the individual to attend meetings and involve himself or herself in the principles and activities of the program. All are invited regardless of race, sex, sexual orientation, social class, health, disability, or personal history.

Without a desire to stop the addictive practice, people are not likely to involve themselves with a Twelve Step program, and its benefit to the client without such a desire may be minimal. On the other hand, because of the inclusiveness of Tradition Two, clinicians can feel comfortable referring any client suffering from addiction or compulsive behavior to a Twelve Step program should the client express a wish for help in that area. Specific types of meetings are allowed for in Tradition Four, and a particular type may be more appropriate for a particular client. (For a review of the types of meetings available, see Chapter 1.) Familiarity with the various types of meeting in one's area will help facilitate an effective referral.

Tradition Four: "Each group should be autonomous except in matters affecting other groups or A.A. as a whole."

With the limited boundaries established in this Tradition—"matters affecting other groups or A.A. as a whole"—authority is released to the group to function in any way it chooses. "Every A.A. group can manage its affairs exactly as it pleases, except when A.A. as a whole is threatened."[9] The only restraints are the welfare of the organization and other groups as determined, again, by group conscience. Thus, specialty groups for women, men, gays and lesbians, physicians, bikers, and other subgroups abound. "Any two or three alcoholics gathered together for sobriety may call themselves an A.A. group provided that as a group they have no other affiliation."[10] If a member does not like a group, he or she can find a few like-minded members and together design a new one. This freedom may result in positive experiences or negative ones from which the members can learn valuable lessons. The founding members of A.A. felt "there was perfect safety in the process of trial and error."[9]

The value of group autonomy is that members have the freedom to establish an ambience in their groups that best fosters their particular needs in staying sober. "Autonomy gives our groups the freedom to act on their own to establish an atmosphere of recovery, serve their members and fulfill their primary purpose."[11] As their individual needs change, members may move from meeting to meeting; groups may dissolve and reform. For example, a new member may initially feel most comfortable in a same-sex meeting. Later, however, this same member, more secure in his or her sobriety, may seek out a more heterogeneous group in which to further his or her process of reconnecting with the world. As mentioned, a clinician well versed in the variety of groups available can assist a client in finding one that is best tailored to his or her particular situation.

Tradition Five: "Each group has but one primary purpose—to carry its message to the alcoholic who still suffers."

Tradition Five speaks to a key characteristic of Twelve Step groups that has helped them maintain their vitality over the years: singleness of purpose. By keeping the focus only on the one thing the program offers—the wisdom of one addict sharing the story of his or her suffering and recovery with another—there is no dilution of energies or confusion over intent. While the Twelve Steps is not an easy program, it is a simple one, and from the beginning the founders felt that it was "better to do one thing supremely well than many badly."[12]

There is another reason, however, for the narrow construction of the Twelve Step mission, one that is more immediate and crucial to the membership. "It is the great paradox of A.A. that we know we can seldom keep the precious gift of sobriety unless we give it away."[13] Members feel that their sobriety—and therefore, their very lives—depends upon having the opportunity to "carry the message" in meetings and Twelfth Step work. The singleness of purpose is for many members only due recognition of the seriousness of the disease with which they struggle. One attends a Twelve Step meeting for one reason: to stay sober by receiving the message and passing it on. For newcomers, Tradition Five provides for clarity and consistency at a time in their lives when little is clear and the very ground may seem to be shifting constantly beneath their feet. Tradition Five keeps the group focus on the survival of the addicts who attend the meetings. This Tradition explicitly defines what clinicians can expect from the program for their clients—no more and no less.

Tradition Six: "An A.A. group ought never endorse, finance, or lend the A.A. name to any related facility or outside enterprise, lest problems of money, property, and prestige divert us from our primary purpose."

Tradition Six provides a list of potential pitfalls that may distract members from the group's purpose as defined by Tradition Five. This "policy of non-affiliation" protects the organization from unwittingly compromising its integrity by not extending its reach beyond that which it can control.[14] Endorsements cannot easily be rescinded; outside organizations may fail to live up to expectations and thereby cause serious public relations damage. Poor outside financial investments by a group would create serious conflict within the group just as certainly as wise outside investments would cast doubt on the motives of the members. Tradition Six aims at warding off potentially fatal distractions to the group's primary reason for being.

Tradition Seven: "Every A.A. group ought to be fully self-supporting, declining outside contributions."

The "principle of corporate poverty" embodied in Tradition Seven serves a variety of purposes: (1) It reiterates the ideas in Tradition Six in that just as groups do not compromise their integrity by investing financially outside the group, neither do they open themselves up to outside control or undue influence from outside contributors which may compromise or distract them from their singleness of purpose. (2) It reinforces the notion of personal accountability and responsibility of the members, the significance of which is evident in the founders' wry comments in *Twelve Steps and Twelve Traditions*—"Self-supporting alcoholics? Who ever heard of such a thing?" (3) It keeps participation in the fellowship essentially free—or at least very inexpensive—and therefore available to anyone regardless of means.[15]

This third factor may be very important for the clinician looking for stable, on-going support for an addict/alcoholic attempting to stay clean and sober. Many addicts, when they reach the stage of "bottoming out" in their disease and finally become willing to seek help, find themselves in precarious or even disastrous financial straits. Twelve Step meetings are, as Tradition Seven states, self-supporting according to the free-will decision of each member to put money in the basket—or not—according to the individual's dictates of conscience. Most members put in one or two dollars each meeting; some donate more, others less, some nothing at all. The basket or hat is passed at each meeting, but no one is forced or even pressured to contribute and no one is ever asked to leave who chooses not to contribute. By keeping expenses at a minimum—donations go to rent, supplies, literature, and to support the General Service Office—Tradition Seven once again emphasizes spiritual priorities over the material.

Tradition Eight: "Alcoholics Anonymous should remain forever nonprofessional, but our service centers may employ special workers."

Tradition Eight repeats the emphasis on the fundamental one-to-one structure of the program. As the *Narcotics Anonymous* text puts it, "We are simply addicts of equal status freely helping one another."[16] This Tradition was originally conceived to prevent members from engaging in Twelfth Step work for financial reward. The founders believed that making money through the program violated the singleness of purpose codified in Tradition Five. The founders feared that as soon as some motivating factor other than the member's desire to stay sober entered in to Twelfth Step work—carrying the message to other alcoholics and addicts—the interpersonal spiritual dynamic that resulted in the miracle of sobriety would be destroyed. Also, by not claiming expertise in anything other than their own experience as hopeless addicts and alcoholics, members do not get drawn in to the scientific or religious controversies of the day. They do not have to promote or defend anything—they just have to tell their stories.

The second part of the Step resolves the controversy over paid staff positions. Someone has to maintain the General and World Service offices. Tradition Eight differentiates between the need for establishing minimal paid administrative and maintenance positions and doing Twelfth Step work. The paid employees are not doing Twelfth Step work, but they do help create the context in which it can be done. Thus, the purpose of both parts of this Tradition—maintaining the nonprofessional stance of members and allowing for administrative staff—is "to make Twelfth Step work possible."[17]

Some clinicians may be threatened by the nonprofessionalism of Twelve Step groups or use that trait to question their validity. However, many clinicians, focused on the best interests and well-being of their clients, will see these groups as a valuable adjunct to the therapeutic process and will choose to incorporate them into their treatment goals.

Tradition Nine: "A.A., as such, ought never be organized; but we may create service boards or committees directly responsible to those they serve."

In an early draft, this Tradition stated that, "Alcoholics Anonymous needs the least possible organization." After some consideration, the founders realized that *no* organization was even better. As there is no organization, there are no membership rules. No one can expel members or dictate to them in any way. Appropriate involvement in the program is insured by disaster: "Unless each A.A. member follows to the best of his ability our suggested Twelve Steps to recovery, he almost certainly signs his own death warrant."[18] The same is presumed true of the groups with the Traditions: groups that do not honor the Traditions will not last. "A.A. has to function, but at the same time it must avoid those dangers of great wealth, prestige, and entrenched power which necessarily tempt other societies."[19] Again, A.A. turns worldly values on their heads by consciously eschewing the very things most organizations actively seek.

One must consider the odds of survival for an "organization" that resists ever being organized. Yet A.A., N.A. and other mutual-help groups based on the Twelve Steps continue to grow and thrive. What seems to hold them together is a combination of humility, radical integrity, and the mystery of honest spiritual inquiry and practice.

Tradition Ten: "Alcoholics Anonymous has no opinion on outside issues; hence the A.A. name ought never be drawn into public controversy."

Again, this Tradition reinforces and further clarifies ideas set forth in previous Traditions, particularly Six and Eight. As mentioned, disengaging from worldly controversies protects the singular focus of the Twelve Step society. In this as in many of the Traditions, the founders used as cautionary tale the history of the Washingtonian Society, a nineteenth century movement of alcoholics many consider a proto-Alcoholics Anonymous. The Washingtonians had a membership in excess of 100,000 at one time, but they became embroiled in the political issues of the day—abolition, temperance, and others—and in their zeal "to reform America's drinking habits ... completely lost their effectiveness in helping alcoholics" stay sober.[20] With their central purpose fatally compromised, the Washingtonian movement soon disappeared. Thus, A.A. and its individual groups hold no official position on any subject, including best practices for chemical dependency treatment, DWI laws, therapeutic modalities, or the criminalization or decriminalization of psychotropic substances. Individually, of course, members may have opinions on any or all of these issues, and many more. But Tradition Ten asks that they not promote these opinions on the authority of their membership in the Twelve Step fellowship.

Tradition Eleven: "Our public relations policy is based on attraction rather than promotion; we need always maintain personal anonymity at the level of the press, radio, and films."

This Tradition does not mean A.A. does not desire coverage in the media or in any way fears such scrutiny. It does, however, seek to discourage any member from speaking for the organization or even for an individual group. "This tradition is a constant and practical reminder that personal ambition has no place in A.A."[21] While Step Twelve admonishes the member to "carry the message," such activity is about offering relief, presenting "a way out" to the suffering addict; it is not about proselytizing because there is no underlying ideology or theology to promote. Again, the singleness of purpose of Twelve Step societies prevents any such thing. "Our public image consists of what we have to offer, a successful proven way of maintaining a drug free lifestyle ... Our attraction is that we are successes in our own right."[16]

Obviously, clinicians must respect this anonymity for their clients. In addition, however, they must realize that no Twelve Step group will come calling or send mail solicitations to promote membership. While members will willingly come to speak to the client about their own experiences and groups will welcome all newcomers who have the desire to stop using, this help must be sought out by the client. The clinician can provide a key role in helping the client to take this step.

Tradition Twelve: "Anonymity is the spiritual foundation of all our Traditions, ever reminding us to place principles above personalities."

Contrary to popular opinion, the principle of anonymity exists less for the protection of the addict or alcoholic from the sanctions of the outside world than to protect the world—and the fellowship itself—from the grandiose thinking of the newly clean and sober member. That is why Tradition Twelve calls it the "spiritual foundation"—its intent is to promote in Twelve Step members an attitude of humility and sacrifice of personal desire for the common good. It is true that originally the impulse behind anonymity was fear of disclosure. The founders quickly discovered, however, that the result of that type of anonymity was a secret society that did not work because no one knew about it. Over the years, anonymity took on a wholly different tenor that focused on the proper stance of the individual in relation to the world rather than the other way around. "We are sure that humility, expressed as anonymity, is the greatest safeguard that Alcoholics Anonymous can ever have."[22]

The *Narcotics Anonymous* text expands on this idea: "Throughout our Traditions we speak in terms of 'we' and 'our' rather than 'me' and 'mine.'"[23] Again, the fellowship is paramount, and no one individual can represent it. The practice of anonymity insures that the focus remains on the principles of the program.

Twelve Step societies are spiritual programs attended by people who have marked difficulties incorporating in their daily affairs such principles as humility, service, sacrifice of personal desires for the greater good, and honesty and integrity. They have found themselves, however, in such dire life circumstances that they are in need of these very principles in order to survive. Twelve Steps programs offer addicts and alcoholics a plan of action to acquire an understanding and develop a practice of these principles. The Twelve Traditions represent both a model of the application of these principles at an organizational level and a protection of the principles themselves from compromise, dilution, and distraction that could destroy the fellowships based upon them.

REFERENCES

1. Ernest Kurtz, *Not-God: A History of Alcoholics Anonymous* (Center City, MN: Hazelden, 1979) p. 111.
2. *The Twelve Steps and Twelve Traditions* (New York: Alcoholics Anonymous World Services, Inc., 1988) p. 133.
3. *The Twelve Steps and Twelve Traditions* (New York: Alcoholics Anonymous World Services, Inc., 1988) p. 134.
4. *The Twelve Steps and Twelve Traditions* (New York: Alcoholics Anonymous World Services, Inc., 1988) p. 138.
5. *Narcotics Anonymous, 5th Ed.* (Van Nuys, CA: N.A. World Services, Inc., 1988) p. 58.
6. *The Twelve Steps and Twelve Traditions* (New York: Alcoholics Anonymous World Services, Inc., 1988) p. 142.
7. *The Twelve Steps and Twelve Traditions*, (New York: Alcoholics Anonymous World Services, Inc., 1988) p. 143.
8. *Narcotics Anonymous, 5th Ed.* (Van Nuys, CA: N.A. World Services, Inc., 1988) p. 59.
9. *The Twelve Steps and Twelve Traditions* (New York: Alcoholics Anonymous World Services, Inc., 1988) p. 150.
10. *The Twelve Steps and Twelve Traditions* (New York: Alcoholics Anonymous World Services, Inc., 1988) p. 151.
11. *Narcotics Anonymous, 5th Ed.* (Van Nuys, CA: N.A. World Services, Inc., 1988) p. 61.
12. *The Twelve Steps and Twelve Traditions* (New York: Alcoholics Anonymous World Services, Inc., 1988) p. 154.
13. *The Twelve Steps and Twelve Traditions* (New York: Alcoholics Anonymous World Services, Inc., 1988) p. 155.

14. *Narcotics Anonymous, 5th Ed.* (Van Nuys, CA: N.A. World Services, Inc., 1988) p. 63.
15. *The Twelve Steps and Twelve Traditions* (New York: Alcoholics Anonymous World Services, Inc., 1988) p. 169, 164.
16. *Narcotics Anonymous, 5th Ed.* (Van Nuys, CA: N.A. World Services, Inc., 1988) p. 68.
17. *The Twelve Steps and Twelve Traditions* (New York: Alcoholics Anonymous World Services, Inc., 1988) p. 172.
18. *The Twelve Steps and Twelve Traditions* (New York: Alcoholics Anonymous World Services, Inc., 1988) p. 178.
19. *The Twelve Steps and Twelve Traditions* (New York: Alcoholics Anonymous World Services, Inc., 1988) p. 179.
20. *The Twelve Steps and Twelve Traditions* (New York: Alcoholics Anonymous World Services, Inc., 1988) p. 183.
21. *The Twelve Steps and Twelve Traditions* (New York: Alcoholics Anonymous World Services, Inc., 1988) p. 187.
22. *The Twelve Steps and Twelve Traditions* (New York: Alcoholics Anonymous World Services, Inc., 1988) p. 192.
23. *Narcotics Anonymous, 5th Ed.* (Van Nuys, CA: N.A. World Services, Inc., 1988) p. 69.

15

Chapter Fifteen

Criticism of the Twelve Steps

The Twelve Steps have been criticized since their inception, but meetings continue to grow and the programs prosper. Two basic levels of criticism exist: first that they are "religious" programs, and second that they are only effective for a small group of people, primarily Christian white males. These criticisms have appeared in the popular lay literature as well as in professional literature. A thorough knowledge of Twelve Step programs as well as an understanding of the Twelve Step subculture and their activities contradicts most of the arguments. Wallace revealed a problem that critics seldom consider: "The extended meanings that characterize the A.A. language system will continue to elude external observers who remain at literal, concrete levels of analysis and fail to consider the nature of symbolic communication and the purposes it serves in complex social contexts and transactions."[1] Without experiencing Twelve Step culture, the professional or lay critic can negatively interpret and even dismiss aspects of these programs that appear to be biased and limited. Yet, immersing oneself into the culture of recovery found in these meetings exposes the healing power of Twelve Step principles. These are mutual help programs, communities of healing. They are not treatment programs that can be governed and altered by the sciences; nonetheless, they are frequently referred to in the critical literature as a form of treatment.

A prime example of this misinterpretation is found in the criticism of the introductory statements used at most Twelve Step meetings; "I'm Dave, and I'm an alcoholic." It is suggested that this statement, used repeatedly, reinforces a negative self-image, that of being an alcoholic. Therapists often use this argument to suggest that Twelve Step programs do not promote growth or individual development, and in fact, hinder members by forcing them to consistently view themselves in such an offensive manner. The Twelve Step perspective is remarkably different. It is believed that public repetition of this accurate statement is necessary to break through denial, develop self-acceptance, and establish a new level of honesty, allowing the individual to begin a Twelve Step recovery program. The terms alcoholic and addict are not understood as negative in these meetings; in fact, they represent positive attributes, identify one as a member of the group, and define involvement in recovery, not active addiction. These become endearing terms, and the introductory statement frankly expresses commitment to a new way of life based on spiritual principles. The uninformed observer is unable to recognize the profound significance of these statements, thus promoting misinformation based on therapeutic principles that are not necessarily relevant to this subculture.

It has never been suggested that the Twelve Steps are for everyone, but there has been tremendous diversification and growth around the world. A.A. meetings are now found in 171 different countries or territories. From the beginning of A.A., the founders meant to be as inclusive as possible in helping anyone who had a problem with alcohol. As A.A. began in the US, the predominant culture (white American male) played a role in preventing certain groups from early involvement, but the very nature of the meetings, based as they are on "group conscience," allowed for groups to adapt to the needs of any special interest. This has transformed A.A. into an extremely diverse organization, with meetings representing most minority groups, subcultures, nations, and religions. K. Makela et al.[2] published a study of A.A. in eight different countries: Austria, Finland, Iceland, Mexico, Poland, Sweden, Switzerland, and the US. They reported that from 1981 through

1990, A.A. grew at a rate 60 percent greater in the rest of the world than in the US (11.5 to 7.2 percent). The same basic structure and core program was noted in the different countries. They did describe some variability in the workings and understanding of the A.A. program, especially in the nature of a Higher Power and the degree of intimacy expressed in group settings.

Major US cities have meetings representing women, men, African Americans, Native Americans, Hispanics, professionals, doctors, nurses, bikers, gays, lesbians, the elderly, adolescents, and other ethnic and interest groups. If Twelve Step programs were only suited for Christian white males, this degree of involvement by remarkably diverse groups and cultures would not have occurred. "The core of the Twelve Steps is spiritual and relative. The truth of this is borne out by the variety of cultures, including those in Eastern Europe and Asia, embodying a wide variety of religious beliefs as well as degrees of atheism and agnosticism, where the Twelve Step movement has taken root and begun to flourish."[3]

Many have been critical of A.A. because it was established as gender specific, by males and for males. For this reason some have suggested that it cannot be appropriate or even useful for women. Some of the cultural biases of the 1930s are reflected in A.A. literature, and early meetings did not include women. One could argue that women were not even considered to be alcoholic during this period in history, but after some initial difficulties with such biases, woman became involved in A.A. The first women's meetings were started in the early 1940s. The *A.A. Grapevine* published the first article addressing the special problems facing women alcoholics in 1945. Thus women play an important role in the history of A.A., and continue to show steady growth and involvement. According to the Alcoholics Anonymous membership survey, women constituted 22 percent of the membership in 1968, 30 percent in 1983, and 35 percent in 1992.[*] It can certainly be difficult for women to read some of the older A.A. literature due

---

[*] Alcoholics Anonymous 1993 Membership Survey, A.A. World Services.

to the gender-specific bias, and if they end up in a male dominated meeting they can feel like outsiders. Nonetheless, the primary aspects of alcoholism affect men and women similarly, the Steps are not gender specific, nor is the experience of recovery.

African Americans have also been active since the early history of A.A. As with women, the dominant cultural biases limited their initial involvement. This prejudice affected some members of A.A., but others recognized that alcoholism crossed all racial and cultural boundaries. Bill Wilson, a cofounder of A.A., was criticized in 1940 for bringing two African Americans to a New York A.A. meeting. His emphasis was to help anyone with alcoholism, and it is this perspective that has been advanced by A.A. and the other Twelve Step programs. African American groups had started in several major US cities by 1945, with general acceptance of African Americans by A.A. as a whole noted by the late 1940s. This is not to say that prejudice has not been a problem, but the A.A. Traditions specifically limit opinions on outside issues, and establish anonymity as a core organizational feature; the literature describes a program based on "principles not personalities." A.A. addresses alcoholism regardless of who has the problem. African Americans have come to accept Twelve Step programs and readily recognize them as effective in addressing alcoholism and addiction. In general, African Americans are very accepting of the spirituality of the Twelve Steps, easing their entry into these recovery programs. Henry Hudson argued that A.A. is effective among African Americans because it provides strong group cohesion and counters the experiences of powerlessness, isolation, and estrangement experienced by many African American alcoholics.[4]

Use of the word "powerless," a necessary concept to recovery in Twelve Step programs (see Chapter 5, Step 1), has generated negative reactions and criticism from feminists and therapists. They have argued that this emphasis is disempowering and undermines those who are already in a powerless position in the dominant culture, especially women and minorities. Step One emphasizes recognition of the problem that the individual is out of control over drugs, alcohol, and the behavior resulting from their chronic use. The admission of powerlessness and unmanageability is a statement of the addict's relationship to the problem. Thus, the criticism does not take into account the condition and needs of the active addict. Addiction is disempowering in a profoundly comprehensive manner. Active addicts find themselves in tragic circumstances, hopeless, despairing, trapped in life-threatening dependence. They need help, but the nature of addiction is to deny the problem, at the very least to deny that one is out of control. It is essential that the addict first recognize the problem: "admitted we were powerless over alcohol." These are not required treatment exercises, but twelve suggested Steps, available to those desperate enough to try them of their own volition. Through the recognition of limitation and the honest examination of consequences the process of recovery can begin. The First Step is a beginning, a foundation upon which to build a new life; its very essence is empowering. "The experience of defeat not only serves to convince the alcoholic that change is necessary; it is the first step in that change ... To be defeated by the bottle and to know it is the first 'spiritual' experience."[5] " 'Not God' means first 'You are not God,' the message of the A.A. program. ... The fundamental and first message of Alcoholics Anonymous to its members is that they are not absolute, not infinite, *not God*. ... But Alcoholics Anonymous is fellowship as well as program, and thus there is a second side to its message of not-God-ness. Because the alcoholic is not God, not absolute, not infinite, he or she is essentially limited. Yet from this very limitation—from the alcoholic's acceptance of personal limitation—arises the beginning of healing and wholeness."[6]

These Steps are based on spiritual principles, which may result in some of the misunderstanding and criticism (see Chapter 2). There is a mistaken belief that one must relinquish all personal power to others or to a Higher Power, perhaps even a paternal god. The Second and Third Steps (see Chapters 6 and 7) provide an expression of the solution to the problem of addiction, but examining them literally, lacking the experience of the participants, can give the impression that the member is being asked to give up complete control of his or her life. The Twelve Step perspective is one of enlisting power from outside oneself, including but not exclusive to the fellowship of other members. Most addicts have experienced innumerable failed attempts to heal themselves and are relieved when they come to the realization that they can rely on the help provided by others and a Higher Power. Receiving the support of others who have gone through the same disasters and are living remarkably different lives can instill hope and provide recognition of a successful route to recovery.

Twelve Step programs are spiritual paths to recovery from addiction. They can only be understood in this context. The ability to do so will enhance the skeptic's comprehension of these remarkable programs. These are spiritual programs that emphasize a personal examination of the individual's beliefs; A.A. is not religion. The initial intent was to use a spiritual approach to address alcoholism but to remain completely separate from religion. The Twelve Steps are not a cult: they do not suggest any specific belief, nor is one asked to dismiss one's own beliefs. In fact, choosing a Higher Power is an essential freedom upon which the program is founded. The Third Step directs the individual to determine their own Higher Power—"God as you understand Him." Although the language suggests a masculine God, the understanding is unlimited and inclusive. The Twelve Steps were written by a group of alcoholic men in the US in the 1930s, many of whom were Christian. For this reason there are references in the A.A. literature that are of Christian origin. The organization does not support nor endorse any religion, and has emphasized the personal expression of a Higher Power, not any particular religion or belief. Unfortunately, some people are unable to consider a program that suggests the use of spirituality, limiting the Twelve Steps as an option. The founders faced this dilemma among their peers. They devoted a chapter of the Big Book to it (Chapter 4, "We Agnostics"), and worked to minimize such problems in order to help as many alcoholics as possible. "When, therefore, we speak to you of God, we mean your conception of God. This applies, too, to other spiritual expressions which you find in this book. Do not let any prejudice you may have against spiritual terms deter you from honestly asking yourself what they mean to you."[7]

Although both the American Medical Association and the American Psychiatric Association have defined alcoholism as a disease, there remains controversy over this issue. Twelve Step programs discuss physical attributes of alcohol and addiction but have never defined alcoholism or addiction. A.A. chose to describe the alcoholic's experience, not to define alcoholism. A.A. has consistently stated that this task is up to the professionals. In spite of this, many critics attribute the terminology "disease concept" or "disease model" to A.A. These terms actually came out of chemical dependency treatment programs, many of which use A.A. principles. *Alcoholics Anonymous* does not use the word disease in referring to alcoholism. The intent of the founders was to provide some basic information about alcoholism based on the founders' own experience so newcomers could better understand their problem. A preface to *Alcoholics Anonymous* entitled "The Doctors Opinion" refers to physical attributes of the alcoholic: "The body of the alcoholic is quite as abnormal as his mind. ... In our belief, any picture of the alcoholic which leaves out this physical factor is incomplete. ... an allergy to alcohol."[8] References about the physical aspects of alcoholism were influenced by William D. Silkworth, who wrote a section of the preface. He was an early supporter of A.A. after witnessing the remarkable changes in alcoholics who engaged in Twelve Step groups. A.A. endorses a physical, psychological and spiritual approach to recovery based on recognition of deterioration of the alcoholic individual in these three spheres.

Several other criticisms about the use of a medical model are attributed to A.A., and will be briefly addressed. Some therapists believe that medical models emphasize the pathological, a negative perspective that can undermine positive self-concept. Once again, A.A. perceives their efforts as positive, providing remarkable support for the newcomer while promoting accurate recognition of the problem. Therapists know that one must separate the addict from the behavior. Addictive disease causes good people to do terrible acts. Twelve Step programs understand this and work to address the guilt and shame people bring with them when they enter early recovery. The disease model of alcoholism has been used as a legal defense suggesting that the inebriate, who is ill, cannot be responsible for his or her own behavior. This is completely counter to Twelve Step philosophy that encourages the members to be fully responsible for past and current behavior. Some professionals still adhere to an old perspective, that alcoholism and addiction are not primary illnesses, but secondary to other emotional problems. This is not supported by the medical definitions, nor by any research, but appears related to old school psychoanalytic theory that has continued to impress certain therapeutic disciplines.

Some people suggest that Twelve Step programs are dependency producing themselves. They refer to them as substitute addictions, or even a pathologic dependency. It is true that some people attend meetings daily and can neglect other aspects of their lives to devote time to recovery. This may be an activity essential to abstinence during the initial phase of recovery. Twelve Step programs do embrace the concept of fellowship, especially in the form of support from other members. "The therapeutic power of this process of identification arose from the witness it gave, a witness to the healing potency of the shared honesty of mutual vulnerability openly acknowledged."[9] Twelve Step programs are based on sharing and connectedness. Meeting attendance and active involvement with others is encouraged. These programs are the antithesis of the isolation of the addictive lifestyle. There is a mutual dependence that can be attributed to such programs, which is no more pathologic than the mutual dependence found among any group of intimate friends. As a general rule, the longer people are abstinent the less they attend meetings. Bill Wilson believed that A.A. is a program to be used to enhance one's life, not to become one's life. People with addictive disease often tend to become addictive (or compulsive) in regard to many other activities, so it is not unusual for them to overdo any number of behaviors in their search for balance. A professional with knowledge of this can act to thwart unhealthy compulsions. Another argument in relation to pathologic dependence suggests that active A.A. involvement results in sobriety, but poor social and psychological adjustment. The research literature does not support this view. Humphreys, Finney, and Moos described more active cognitive and behavioral coping, less avoidant coping, and more social support from friends, among people with greater A.A. involvement.[10] A.A. involvement was also reported to have a positive correlation with improved psychological adjustment by Emrick et al. [11]

Abstinence itself is considered too rigorous by certain groups, which fault Twelve Step programs for their approach. Most of these criticisms refer to A.A. as treatment, or are directed at Twelve Step oriented treatment programs. The general arguments are that some people cannot maintain abstinence, others should not be made to feel like failures if they do not meet the goal of abstinence, and others can be treated with a harm reduction approach that does not require abstinence. Twelve Step programs do not have opinions on these "outside issues." What they do provide is a program with a simple approach: "the only requirement for membership is a desire to stop drinking."[13] Most members of A.A. would consider it irrational and absurd for an alcoholic to attempt controlled drinking for they understand alcoholism as an inability to control alcohol use, powerlessness. The foundation of Twelve Step programs, which provides for the remarkable life changes experienced by those who work these spiritual programs of recovery, is abstinence. Furthermore, abstinence is not enough for A.A. members—the goal is to advance one's life spiritually.

One critique that reveals the ignorance and audacity of some mental health professionals is that Twelve Step programs are non-professional. This is a bias that suggests people with these problems are unable to help one another and that the only group capable of providing care, relief, even a "cure," are properly trained mental health professionals. It is true that Twelve Step programs are not professional, and they are not treatment programs. Twelve Step programs are mutual help programs, and have been tremendously effective without the participation of mental health professionals.

One final note on criticism of Twelve Step programs for the referring professional: those who attend or are asked to attend such programs and who have no interest in abstinence and no desire to stop drinking or using drugs will develop innumerable reasons for avoiding meetings. This will provide the professional with another list of criticisms. Such clients may invoke some of the above mentioned issues as reasons not to attend Twelve Step meetings. It is important for the professional to be able to address these criticisms with some degree of authority, and to witness attempts at manipulation. Do not underestimate the persuasive ability of an addict intent on avoiding a recovery program.

Twelve Step programs are not for everyone. Some of the problems noted in the criticisms outlined in this chapter have kept people away from these meetings. The intent of Twelve Step programs is to help as many people as possible. They are mutual help programs that are very successful, but have a singleness of purpose: for A.A., this is to "solve their common problem and help others to recover from alcoholism."[9] The advancement of these programs, especially A.A., around the world, in remarkably diverse cultures, reveals that the intent of the founders to develop an inclusive program to help alcoholics has succeeded in dramatic fashion. Meetings reflect the attendees, and can be adapted to meet the needs of nearly any special interest group. This has established a formula for continued growth and advancement of a simple program based on spiritual principles.

REFERENCES

1. J. Wallace, Ideology, belief, and behavior: Alcoholics Anonymous as a social movement, in E. Gottheil, K. Draley, T. Skolada, and H. Waxman, eds., *Etiologic Aspects of Alcohol and Drug Use* (Springfield, IL: Charles C. Thomas, 1983) pp. 285–305.
2. K. Makela, I. Arminen, K. Bloomfeild et al., *Alcoholics Anonymous as a Mutual Help Movement* (Madison, WI: University of Wisconsin Press, 1996).
3. David E. Smith, Millicent E. Buxton, Rafiq Bilal, and Richard E. Seymour, Chapter 3, Cultural points of resistance to Twelve step program recovery, in *Principles of Addiction Medicine, 1st Ed.*

(Chevy Chase, MD: American Society of Addiction Medicine, 1994).

4. Henry Hudson, How and why Alcoholics Anonymous works for Blacks, in F. Brisbane and M. Womble, eds., *Treatment of Black Alcoholics* (New York: Hayworth Press, 1985).

5. G. Bateson, *Steps to an Ecology of Mind* (New York: Ballantine, 1972) p. 313.

6. Ernest Kurtz, *Not-God: A History of Alcoholics Anonymous* (Center City, MN: Hazelden, 1979) pp. 3–4.

7. *Alcoholics Anonymous* (New York: Alcoholics Anonymous World Services, Inc., 1976) p. 47.

8. *Alcoholics Anonymous* (New York: Alcoholics Anonymous World Services, Inc., 1976) p. xxiv.

9. Ernest Kurtz, *Not-God: A History of Alcoholics Anonymous* (Center City, MN: Hazelden, 1979) p. 61.

10. K. Humphreys, J.W. Finney, R.H. Moos, Applying a stress and coping framework to research on mutual help organizations, *Journal of Community Psychology*, 1994, 22: 312–327.

11. C.D. Emrick, J.S. Tonigan, H. Montgomery, and L. Little, Alcoholics Anonymous: What is currently known?, in B.S. McCrady and W. R. Miller, eds., *Research on Alcoholics Anonymous: Opportunities and Alternatives* (New Brunswick, NJ: Rutgers Center for *Alcohol Studies*, 1993) pp. 41–76.

12. *Alcoholics Anonymous Preamble*, A.A. Grapevine, 1947.

16

Chapter Sixteen

The Courage to Change:
The Twelve Steps in Action

Working with addicts and alcoholics is extraordinarily gratifying. When they commit to a recovery program the positive changes are dramatic. Clinicians witness the rebuilding of lives and families. It is a privilege to play a role in such a transformation. Members of Twelve Step programs appear to make the most remarkable changes and are the most likely to extend themselves to help others.

Many clinicians only witness the worst aspects of addiction and do not observe this transformation. They see trauma victims in emergency rooms, some of them intoxicated, others with injuries caused by the intoxicated. They try to stem the tide of acute illness directly related to the addiction. They deal with abuse, neglect, psychosis, and self-destructiveness. They treat many of these clients repeatedly. They work with families that are disintegrating, despairing children, and frantic husband and wives. Therapists may identify the problem, but in so doing loose the client. For many clinicians, the miracle of recovery is but a myth. They only see the tragedy, which reinforces the perception that these people are loathsome, undisciplined and untreatable. They do not believe this is a disease, have only witnessed failure, and quit trying to make a difference. Unfortunately, the addict stuck in the cycle of addiction is of a similar opinion, perhaps even more thoroughly convinced, and has great difficulty seeking help. Addicts often do not even believe they deserve help. Members of

Twelve Step programs know these feelings well. They have lived through the tragedy and know the true miracles of recovery. They are often the only ones who can reach the addicted person, and feel obligated to do so, knowing it will help themselves to carry the message. They can provide hope in human form with their stories of recovery.

Cindy is a twenty-five-year-old member of A.A. She had been using methamphetamine and alcohol in an addictive manner from age sixteen until she entered treatment at twenty-two. She ran away from home and dropped out of high school. She rejected her family, and did not stay in contact with them after leaving. She has been married and divorced twice, the first to the father of her two older daughters. Their divorce was secondary to her inability to stop using drugs and alcohol. The second was to a very physically and sexually abusive methamphetamine addict that threatened to kill her if she ever turned him in or left him. They had a two-year-old daughter. Due to her addiction the two older daughters were removed from her care by the state and placed with their father. The state had custody of the youngest daughter, and had placed her with a foster family, allowing Cindy supervised visits once a week, which she often missed. Her addiction was severe, she had no substantial income, and she was only able to leave her violent ex-husband by going to a battered women's shelter. She was frightened, disgraced, ashamed of herself, and barely able to admit to herself that her daughters had been taken from her care. She was significantly underweight and malnourished, had a severe urinary tract infection, multiple bruises, and was extremely disheveled. For the first time in her life she was ready to ask for help.

The shelter staff arranged for her to enter a treatment program, and she began to care for herself again. While there she was exposed to the Twelve Steps and had a chance to attend A.A. She was immediately attracted to the members of the group she attended and found herself accepted in a manner she had not experienced in adulthood. She had yet to begin to like herself—at times she despised herself for what she had done—but these people seemed genuinely appreciative of her involvement in their group. She felt at home among the alcoholics and addicts who so willingly told her their own tragic stories and suggested she call them if she needed to talk. At first she did not feel deserving of taking someone's time by calling them but later began to do so. She was fascinated by several of the other women who could so easily describe the calamity of their past, even laugh about it, and seemed genuinely happy with their current lives. Sometimes she had difficulty believing they had ever been like her, but the stories were too familiar and painful to be fabricated. She chose a sponsor after a long period of agonizing over having to let someone into her life. The woman had many of the same experiences as Cindy and readily understood many of her problems. She often provided stories from her own experience or a reminder of a Step to consider when facing certain problems, but she never told Cindy what to do, allowing her to make her own decisions. Cindy felt loved by her sponsor and some of the other group members. This allowed her to begin to feel as if maybe she was worthwhile, perhaps even lovable. She cried about her children frequently and her sponsor told her to "let go," use the Serenity Prayer, and pray for them to get what they needed. At first she did not understand how this approach could help at all; she wanted to be their mother. Over time she realized that she needed to concentrate on recovery, on taking care of herself, so that she could become the woman and mother she was meant to be.

Cindy had completed the first five Steps while in treatment, and shared them with her sponsor who had something special to add to each that had not been mentioned or discussed in the treatment program. She found it easy to accept the First Step—she was desperate to change her life. She had been raised in a religious household but had rejected belief in a God while she was using drugs and being abused. In spite of this, the spiritual approach appealed to her. She wanted to believe in a Power for good, a Power that would help her just as it had her new found friends. She developed a strong belief, then started to consider her Higher Power's role in her daily life. This was unlike any attempt she had ever made at understanding how to lead her life, yet it appealed to her. She had followed her own path of self-destruction and really did not trust herself to find the way out alone. The Fourth Step was difficult for Cindy. She did not want to examine certain aspects of her past, and still could not believe that she had chosen drugs over her own children. She was a bit confused by how to address the abuse, but settled on a way of examining her own life, sticking to a personal inventory, and avoiding the trap of blaming her problems on circumstances. She decided to enter into psychotherapy to specifically address the abuse. This allowed her to focus on her own behavior in the Fourth Step, while using her therapist to address the victimization, fear, and lack of trust that skewed her relationships. She wanted to change and repeatedly made decisions to do whatever was necessary. The Fifth Step resulted in a sense of freedom unlike anything she had ever experienced. She truly felt as if she had left some of the shame and guilt behind, and was able to move forward without constantly doubting and berating herself. She took responsibility for what she had done to her children and found this allowed her to begin the process of healing these relationships.

Cindy was ready for the Sixth and Seventh Steps. She had come to understand that her recovery was not just about staying sober—she wanted a better life. Her commitment to change and the love she had for her children enabled her to consider her defects then ask her higher Power to remove them. She also did the work she knew was necessary to continue the process of self-improvement. She started parenting classes and began to contact her children regularly. This allowed her to start the Eighth and Ninth Steps, not just apologizing, but making amends by leading a life she was proud of, especially regarding re-involvement with her daughters. Without the weight of her own shame, she found the ability to approach the courts, her family, and her ex-husband to demonstrate the progress she had made and to petition them to allow her to be a mother once again.

Cindy now has custody of her youngest daughter and has reestablished a relationship with her ex-husband that has allowed her to spend time with her older daughters on a regular basis. She is attending college part time, while working full time. She continues to attend A.A. twice a week and sponsors two women her own age. She uses a daily inventory to keep close track of herself, and to be certain that she does not backslide. Maintaining conscious contact with her Higher Power has become one of the most important aspects of her life. She has developed spiritual discipline, monitors her thoughts and behaviors, and attempts to express herself with love in all her endeavors. Cindy has experienced the joy associated with the Twelfth Step by committing to lead the best life that she can, which includes a great deal of work with others. She remembers those who helped her so freely, and so she regularly volunteers at a women's shelter and gives talks to local high schools about the calamity of addiction and her experiences with the miracles of recovery. It is a great deal of work: she is not always happy, sometimes lacks confidence, and still makes mistakes. Some of her toughest lessons have come in romantic relationships, and she admits that she has a lot to learn about love. Nonetheless, she is going in the right direction. She is clean and sober, and has discovered a way of life that has restored her self-esteem and given her hope. She believes that the Twelve Steps have provided much more than sobriety, that she is on a spiritual path to healing and wholeness.

Ed is seventy-five, attends A.A. meetings once a week, and has been sober for the past thirty years. He continues to work the Steps, primarily the maintenance Steps, and can spontaneously speak about any of them with authority. People are immediately attracted to this enormous bald man when he begins to describe his thoughts on spirituality and love. With his booming voice, it is almost as if God is speaking. He recognizes the seriousness of this disease from his own experience and twenty years as a chemical dependency counselor. He is regularly asked to speak at A.A. functions and gives sermons at several local churches. He has exceptional knowledge of recovery and the Twelve Steps, as well as religion and the Course in Miracles. He does not limit discussions to A.A., and honors the inclusive, spiritual nature of Twelve Step programs. He is as likely to call a fellow member a bullshitter as he is to speak about the glory of God. When necessary, he describes his own battle with alcohol, but most of his time is spent expressing the richness of a life based on these simple Steps. He references poems as easily as he does A.A. material, and the main reason people listen is that he speaks from his heart to all of us, with a sincerity founded on humility earned through his struggles with alcoholism and the A.A. program. His contribution to the A.A. community is especially noted in the lives of the younger men he has guided and mentored. He is not as active as some, and does little in the way of sponsoring individuals. His gift is in the form of spiritual wisdom, which he exudes, and which people find themselves automatically attempting to emulate. Ed lives the program in such a remarkable way that his presence compels others to grasp it.

Tim is a physician who started A.A. as a high school dropout. He has been sober for the past 24 years. He began A.A. after using drugs and alcohol from age twelve to nineteen. At seventeen he was placed in a treatment program by his parents. He was able to recognize that he had a problem, and admitted to being an addict, but was unable to do anything about it until he entered A.A. over a year later. He describes a series of miracles that completely altered his life course, beginning with A.A. and the opportunity to work in a cardiovascular research lab. He had applied to be a janitor at the medical center, but was hired to be a lab technician. He was attending A.A. and working the Steps when the doctors in the lab began to suggest he attend college. He had no real plans for his future; in fact, prior to entering A.A. had been under the assumption that he would not survive long enough to warrant a college education. He was trying to stay sober and learn the Steps to lead a life based on their principles. He had little in the way of self-confidence but found that he prospered when he worked the Steps and relied on a Higher Power. He began to consider becoming a surgeon, like many of the physicians he worked with. He was hesitant to mention this to anyone, but told his sponsor, who knew him as a young member of A.A. and a high school dropout. His sponsor told him that if it was God's will he would certainly be able to become a doctor. Tim started to pray for guidance, and for the knowledge of God's will, supported, not doubted by his sponsor.

Tim was accepted into college and began on the anniversary of his first year of sobriety. School was very difficult; during drug and alcohol use he had made a distinct attempt to ruin his memory and forget as much about his life as possible. Now he had to rebuild his memory. He had been kicked out of his family's home due to his addiction, and returned for the first time in two years at Christmas after his first semester. His grades were sent to the home and arrived during his stay, revealing that he had made the dean's list. It was an opportunity to share some success rather than tragedy with his family, to make amends, and to register evidence that his new way of life, working a Twelve Step program, was having a positive impact. He attended A.A. on campus, and continued to work the Steps. His abstinence was not fully understood by his friends at school, but they supported him after hearing his story, recognizing that he had an inability to control alcohol or drug use. He began to enjoy learning and blossomed in an academic environment. His attitude about medical school remained consistent with his sponsor's advice—if it was God's will, it would happen. This allowed him to focus on his own responsibility by doing what he could without worrying about the outcome, sure that he would be well taken care of. He used the Serenity Prayer regularly in order to keep his mind on the task at hand, accomplish what he could, and leave the results in God's hands.

Tim was accepted to medical school, but required a major lesson about surrender and God's will. He was devoted to a spiritual path, but began to believe he knew what his Higher Power had in store for him, so he chose not to take a course necessary for one of the schools he had applied to, the one that was most likely to accept him. He was convinced he would get into the school of his choice, the one he was sure God had chosen as well. It did not happen, however; he was accepted at the other school. He was on the waiting list for the desired school, but was not able to count on acceptance. He was extremely upset about the situation, still convinced that he somehow knew what was best for himself. He had plans to work for the summer, and make money for medical school, but now he could not, as he had to take the class he had neglected. It was not available at his university, nor at the medical school. He finally found the required course at a school about thirty miles from his brother's house. He moved in with his brother, used his brother's car, and started the class. Nothing was going as he had planned. Throughout the first day of lectures he was preoccupied with thoughts about his predicament, still angry about the fact that he did not get his way. On the second day of class he began to pray, recognizing that he no longer had a choice and had to complete this course to begin medical school where he had been admitted. He was able to resolve his anger and accept that his will and ideas were not God's will; he began to realize he had no way of knowing what his Higher Power had planned for him. Ultimately he surrendered, accepted his fate, and thanked his Higher Power for the opportunity to go to medical school, realizing that it had taken a series of miracles to even get to this point. He experienced an overwhelming sense of acceptance, recognized that he did not have the ability to predict God's will, and began to focus on the course at hand. That night at his brother's house he received a phone call announcing his acceptance to the school he had been counting on. It was a dramatic, valuable lesson in surrender, and poignantly demonstrated that a Higher Power is in charge and plays a powerful role in his daily life.

Tim went on to complete medical school and specialty training. He would rather discuss great spiritual lessons than his academic and professional accomplishments, but describing the combination has been of great benefit to others in Twelve Step programs. He continues to attend A.A. on a regular basis, and dedicates some of his professional activities to working with alcoholics and addicts. His main goal is to lead a spiritual existence founded in daily discipline and the expression of love.

These are three examples of the remarkable results that can be experienced when members commit to a Twelve Step program. Individuals enter such programs with the intent to address their addiction. "The only requirement for membership is a desire to stop drinking."[1] What they find is considered a joke among members; you have to change your whole life. The goal is to remain abstinent and consistently grow and develop spiritually while living the principles. It is a way of life, not just a way to stay sober. The risk associated with a half-hearted approach is tremendous; the possibility of backsliding into the calamity of addiction, perhaps even death. The stunning results of Twelve Step programs are provided by a nonprofessional fellowship that employs mutual help, without experts, to address an atrocious, baffling disease. Twelve Step programs provide a sanctuary for the addicted, where dedicated members offer acceptance and hope based on their own experience with a spiritual program. Strength flows from acceptance and the open acknowledgment of limitation, furnishing the members with a spiritual path to healing and, ultimately, fulfillment. Twelve Step programs offer clinicians ready access to this successful, inexpensive, inclusive method of addressing addictions based on spiritual principles. Clinicians can use these spiritual principles to support their clients attempts at abstinence, and, once this is established, enhance their transformation. By doing so they can actively participate in the miracles of recovery that result from this simple program.

> The great fact is just this and nothing less: That we have had deep and effective spiritual experiences which have revolutionized our whole attitude toward life, toward our fellows and toward God's universe. The central fact of our lives today is the absolute certainty that our Creator has entered into our hearts and lives in a way that is indeed miraculous. He has commenced to accomplish those things for us which we could never do for ourselves.[2]

REFERENCES

1. *Alcoholics Anonymous Preamble*, A.A. Grapevine, 1947.
2. *Alcoholics Anonymous* (New York: Alcoholics Anonymous World Services, Inc., 1976) p. 25.

1

Appendix 1

Location of A.A. Groups or Loners

AFRICA

Angola/Benin/Botswana/Cape Verde/Egypt/Ethiopia/Ghana/
Kenya/Libya/Madagascar/Malawi/Mali/Mauritius/Morocco/
Mozambique/Namibia/Niger/Nigeria/Réunion/Senegal/Sierra
Leone/South Africa/Swaziland/Tanzania/Uganda/Zaire/Zambia/
Zimbabwe

ASIA & INDIAN OCEAN ISLANDS

Bangladesh/Burma/Cambodia/Diego Garcia/Hong Kong/India/
Indonesia/Japan/Korea/Laos/Malaysia/Nepal/Pakistan/
People's Republic of China/Philippines/Republic of Singapore/
Sri Lanka/Taiwan/Thailand/Vietnam

AUSTRALIA, NEW ZEALAND, PACIFIC ISLANDS & ANTARCTICA

American Samoa/Australia/Cook Islands/Fiji/Guam/Johnston
Island/Marshall Islands/Micronesia/New Caledonia/New
Zealand/Papua New Guinea/Saipan/Solomon Islands/Tahiti/
Tonga/Vanuatu/Western Samoa

BERMUDA & CARIBBEAN ISLANDS

Anguilla/Antigua/Aruba/Bahamas/Barbados/Bermuda/Bonaire/
Cayman Islands/Cuba/Curaçao/Dominica/Dominican Republic/
Grenada/Haiti/Jamaica/Montserrat/Nevis/Saba Island/St.
Barthelemy/St. Kitts/St. Lucia/St. Maarten/St. Vincent/Tortola/
Trinidad and Tobago/Turks and Caicos Islands/Virgin Gorda/
(U.S.) Virgin Islands

EUROPE

Austria/Belarus/Belgium/Bosnia-Herzegovina/Bulgaria/Channel
Islands/Croatia/Czech Republic/Denmark/England/Estonia/
Faroe Islands/Finland/France/Georgia/Germany/Gibraltar/
Greece/Hungary/Iceland/Ireland/Italy/Kazakhstan/Latvia/
Lithuania/Luxembourg/Macedonia/Malta/Moldova/Monaco/
Netherlands/Norway/Poland/Portugal/Romania/Russia/
Scotland/Slovakia/Slovenia/Spain/Sweden/Switzerland/
Ukraine/Wales

MEXICO & CENTRAL AMERICA

Belize/Costa Rica/El Salvador/Guatemala/Honduras/Mexico/
Nicaragua/Panama

NEAR & MIDDLE EAST

Bahrain/Brunei/Cyprus/Israel/Kuwait/Lebanon/Oman/Qatar/
Saudi Arabia/Turkey/United Arab Emirates/Yemen Arab
Republic

NORTH AMERICA

Canada/Greenland/United States

SOUTH AMERICA & FALKLAND ISLANDS

Argentina/Bolivia/Brazil/Chile/Colombia/Ecuador/Guyana/
Paraguay/Peru/Uruguay/Venezuela

2

The Twelve Steps on the World Wide Web

AA Grapevine: http://www.aagrapevine.org

AA History and Trivia: http://www.aahistory.com

AA Online@aol: http://aaonline.net

Adult Children of Alcoholics World Services Organization, Inc.: http://adultchildren.org

Al-Anon and Alateen: http://www.12step-recovery.org

Alcoholics in Recovery: http://Geocities.com/HotSprings/Spa/1799

Alcoholics Anonymous World Services:http://www.alcoholics-anonymous.org

"Another Empty Bottle": http://www.alcoholismhelp.com

The Awareness Center (Adult Children of Alcoholics): http://www.drjan.com

Big Book Concordance: http://royy.com/concord.html

Caron Foundation: http://www.caron.org

Cocaine Anonymous World Services: http://www.ca.org

Codependents Anonymous (CoDA): http://www.codependents.org

Debtors Anonymous: www.debtorsanonymous.org

Gamblers Anonymous: www.gamblersanonymous.org

"Grant Me the Serenity: Self-Help and Recovery": http://www.open-mind.org

Help in Finding a Meeting: http://12stepmeeting.com

Hazelden Foundation: http://www.hazelden.org

"Hope and Healing Web Chronicles": http://www.hopeandhealing.com

Habit Smart: Information about Addictive Behavior: http://www.cts.com/crash/habtsmrt/

Links to Recovery: http://www.webcrafts-by-laura.com/recovery.htm

Marijuana Anonymous World Services: http://dualrecovery.-base.org

Narcotics Anonymous: http://www.na.org

Nicotine Anonymous: http://www.nicotine-anonymous.org

Online AA Recovery Resources: http://www.recovery.org

Overeaters Anonymous: http://www.overeaters.org

Recoveries Anonymous: http://www.r-a.org

Secular Organizations for Sobriety (SOS): http://www.secularhumanism.org/sos/

Sex Addicts Anonymous: http://www.sexaa.org

Sober Dykes Hope Page: http://www.soberdykes.org

Sober Vacations International: http://www.sobervacations.com/index.htm

Sobriety and Recovery Resources: http://www.recoveryresources.org

Substance Abuse Issues: http://www.jointogether.org

"12 Step Cyber Café": http://www.12steps.com

Twelve Step Meetings, National and International: http://12stepmeetings.com/index.html

Index